D1520711

The HIDDEN CONNECTION

Discover What's Keeping You from Feeling Happy, Healthy and Symptom-free

Kathleen DiChiara, FDN, CHC

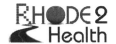

RHODE 2
Health

Copyright © 2014 by Kathleen DiChiara

All rights reserved.

Except as permitted under the U.S. Copyright Act of 1976, no part of this book may be reproduced, distributed, or transmitted in any form or by any means, electronic or mechanical, including photocopying, or by any information storage and retrieval system without the written permission from Rhode to Health Publications.

Rhode to Health
2019 Smith Street
North Providence, RI 02911

Visit our website www.rhodetohealth.com

Printed in the United States of America

First Edition: October 2014

ISBN 978-0-9908223-1-8
$19.95 Softcover

Library of Congress Control Number: 2014918057

The information in this book is for educational purposes only. It is not intended to provide medical advice or to take the place of medical advice and treatment from your personal physician. The reader should always consult their own doctors or other qualified health professionals regarding the treatment of medical conditions including the appropriateness of the information for their own situation. The author shall not be held liable or responsible for any misunderstanding or misuse of the information contained in this book or for any loss, damage, or injury caused or alleged to be caused directly or indirectly by any treatment, action, or application of any food or food source discussed in this book. The statements in this book have not been evaluated by the U.S. Food and Drug Administration. This information is not intended to diagnose, treat, or cure any disease.

Dedication

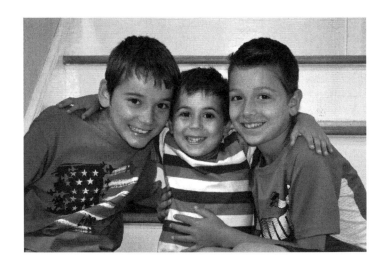

To my three amazing boys:

Stephen, Camden and Treyson

Ironically, my disease became my gift to you.
Without it, I would have missed the opportunity
to teach you the foundation of health
and the importance of living your best life!
Cheers! To breaking the vicious cycle.

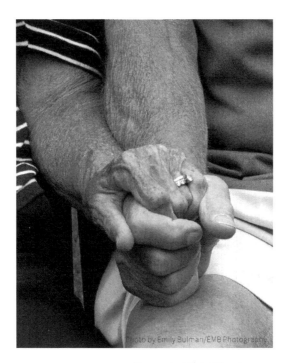

My parents at their 50th anniversary.

GRATITUDE

A BOOK IS NEVER WRITTEN IN A VACUUM. TO ALL OF THE PEOPLE
WHO MADE THIS BOOK A REALITY BY SHARING THEIR STRUGGLES WITH
ME AND MOTIVATING ME TO SHARE MY STORY AND KNOWLEDGE ON
A BROADER PLATFORM, I AM DEEPLY GRATEFUL. YOUR STORIES LIVE IN
MY HEART AND ARE CONTAINED ON THE PAGES OF THIS BOOK.

Deep gratitude to my teachers and guides, Joshua Rosenthal and Lindsey Smith, who provided unwavering support and guidance throughout the writing and publishing process. This book was living inside me for years and they provided the framework to bring it to paper and beyond.

A special thanks to Suzanne Boothby who gave me the space, support, guidance and encouragement to dig deeper into my message of hope for others and to write from the heart. Stasia Blanco, my graphic designer, who applied her passion and skills to transform my words and information into visual art—I am so grateful.

To my mom and dad who gave me a strong foundation of family values that carry into my family life today, like eating meals together as a family to stay connected, encouraging free play versus over-scheduled organized play, hard work and dedication, and for modeling unconditional love for each other.

To my sister, Anne Marie, who has demonstrated the courage and determination of a true warrior to battle the "beast" of autoimmune. She is my hero and a constant source of motivation for her willingness to press on and live her best life.

And finally, my deepest gratitude to my husband, Stephen, for his endless love and support. Stephen is my sounding board for ideas often encouraging my explorations while providing a much needed reality check. He is the one person who recognizes my desire to charge on despite my limitations and often reminds me of the importance of pulling back the reigns to return to self care. He provides the stability and humor to our long days (and short years) of raising a family.

Foreword

by Julie Matthews, B.S., N.C.

Something fundamental is missing from the way we care for our health these days.

We have more lifesaving and highly advanced medical technology, yet we have more adults and children suffering chronic diseases than ever before. Our modern world's fast-paced lifestyle, nutrient devoid convenient foods, countless chemical/toxic exposures, and environment stressors are interfering with our cellular function and biology. It's no wonder people are sick.

Despite our advancements, what seems to be missing from the healthcare equation is concerted attention to the quality of things that we put into our bodies every day. That is, the food and nutrition we receive—our diet. The very thing we can control.

The care of health must explore how our biological systems work, the role of nutrition, and how deficiencies and other factors contribute to the epidemic of chronic disease we see today. Nutrition is powerful. It is a piece of the health puzzle that cannot be replaced with quick fixes or a magic bullet.

Fueled by a passion to heal herself and her own children, Kathleen DiChiara has discovered powerful knowledge. In *The Hidden Connection,* she shares her inspiring life-changing journey. As a mom, she studied and learned what all holistic health professionals know; that we are born with a certain genetic code, but that nutrition and environment throughout our lifetime can and do play an even more important role to our physical wellbeing. Nutrition can turn genes "on" or "off," as well as boost impaired biochemical pathways and help restore damaged systems. Conversely, nutrient deficiencies and toxins impair us further by fueling the flame of underlying inflammation. As Kathleen so aptly explains, this is at the core of the unhealthiness and disease rampant in society.

For fourteen years I have specialized in helping families and children with autism. As a Certified Nutrition Consultant, I have worked one on one with hundreds of people in similar situations to Kathleen's.

Sadly, people are routinely given devastating prognoses when facing disorders like autism, PDD, and other chronic diseases. They are often told that a child with autism will never speak, will be in an institution, will not have any friends, and will never say "I love you." I've seen all of these scenarios disproven time and time again when parents empower themselves, change their family's diet, and look for answers.

I want you to know that there is always hope. Don't let anyone tell you otherwise. Find someone who believes in you: a practitioner or a mentor. The very act of increasing your knowledge and fine-tuning your attention to this area of healthcare is beneficial. That is why the essence of my nutritional practice, and book, is *nourishing hope.*

I have seen children's eczema, dark eye circles, runny noses, diarrhea and bloating disappear. I've witnessed children become more social, engaged with the family, sleep better, have improved mood, and increased language. There are many stories around the world of children even fully recovering from autism, losing their diagnosis—something the mainstream model of care does not accept as a possibility. These are not the one-off exceptions; I hear this frequently.

In *The Hidden Connection,* Kathleen shares her four-step D.E.A.P. approach to help guide readers on their unique journey to wellness—to conquer chronic disease, not just manage it. When you learn, as Kathleen says "how to think, not what to think," a world of possibility will open up.

Kathleen's journey exemplifies what I mean by nourishing hope. She had a deep and personal healthcare need that was unaddressed by mainstream thinking, and instead of being deterred, she embraced hope and chose to take matters into her own hands— by becoming intently strategic about dietary choices. She investigated the disordered systems of the body, sought causes and influences of their functioning, and employed sound science and personal experience to discern and apply the bio-individual approach needed to facilitate healing.

It's important to recognize that you cannot always follow someone else's path. You must pave your own way, learning what foods, nutrients, and supplements are best for you. There is no "one size fits all" diet or approach to healing. If one diet or method does not seem to help, explore further. Ultimately, everyone needs good nutrition and a customized approach.

In *The Hidden Connection,* Kathleen shares vital insight with you. She blends lessons learned during her own journey with insight gleaned through professional study in nutrition and health coaching. This book will help you discover new things about your body and it's interconnection with food and the environment, while providing you with an approach that embraces your own journey to wellbeing.

Julie Matthews, B.S., N.C.
Author of *Nourishing Hope for Autism*
Co-founder of BioIndividual Nutrition Institute

Contents

A Message to My Reader

I do not claim to have all the answers. In fact, the more I learn about the human body, the more I am convinced we will never fully understand its magnificence. It is so important for me to let you know just how much I care about you and your personal story. Just because I will be sharing reachable goals and successes in my life, by no means is it intended to minimize your struggle.

If your story doesn't end the way you hoped please know that any attempt to improve your health is always worth it. That is how you learn and grow. That is how you discover things about yourself that you value and cherish. It's an exploration into what I believe is the most important question you can ask yourself—Am I truly living my best life? When you recognize that achieving a healthy body and mind is simply a tool to achieve your biggest dreams in life you can begin to see it (diet) as an ever-changing and dynamic way to honor your unique bio-individual life.

Thank you for the opportunity to serve as your guide. May you find at least one small seed of insight and feel inspired to make this the beginning or extension of your healing journey.

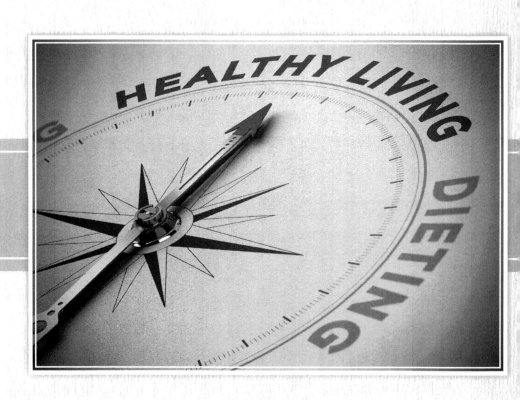

INTRODUCTION

You are trapped inside a body that is malfunctioning and no diet is going to change that. Dieting is not a cure for chronic disease, obesity, or autoimmune disorders. A healthy lifestyle is not about good foods, bad foods. It is about discovering what foods are right for you and what foods are making you sick. And more importantly, a healthy life always goes beyond the plate.

My story

I had a successful career at a Fortune 500 Company that I loved. I married the man of my dreams and had two adorable little boys. We had just bought a new house. Life was good.

It was the summer of 2007 when my life took a dramatic change in course. Despite my commitment to health and fitness, my physical body decided to quit. While I thought I was doing all the "right" things—exercising daily, competing in recreational triathlons, eating whole grains and low fat foods—I was shocked when I woke up one August morning with sudden onset neuropathy in my left leg. In the days just prior I did have low back pain but I quickly attributed this to moving furniture and the stress that accompanies any life transitions, like moving. I expected 'this too shall pass.' Sadly, it didn't. Five short months later, I fell victim to the medical (sick-care) system of surgery, pharmaceuticals, and multiple diagnoses, which left me permanently disabled.

In early 2008, I underwent a fairly standard back surgery (an L4/L5 laminectomy and discectomy). This means the surgeon would shave a portion of my vertebrae bone and the herniated disc with the goal of relieving the compressed nerve causing pain and numbness in the left leg. However, when I woke from my back surgery, I knew something was terribly wrong. My legs wouldn't move. My physical body wasn't working properly; I was scared.

The number of symptoms continued to grow— the paralysis led to chronic pain; my irritable bowel syndrome led to unhealthy weight loss. I was covered in skin rashes, had daily headaches, and remained awake most nights with restless leg syndrome. My restricted movements were matched with weakness and numbness. Eventually my vision became blurred, dizziness set in and I was consumed with chronic fatigue. I was eventually diagnosed with fibromyalgia, degenerative facet joint syndrome, a spinal hemangioma, another disc herniation (this time in my neck), neuropathy, and chronic pain syndrome. And if that wasn't enough, I was now 'allergic' to everything.

As my condition continued to spiral out of control, I felt frustrated and confused. I desperately searched for answers, traveling to the best specialists and considering any and every therapy available. Sadly, the solutions I was offered by medical experts were pills, more surgeries, and treatments to "manage" the pain and symptoms.

I was forced to leave the job I loved because of the uncertainty of my prognosis. I was loosing control of everything I had worked so hard for—my physically fit body, my career and my role as wife and mother.

. . .

So, why did I develop this sudden neuropathy? And, why did my body react so poorly to surgery? Looking back it wasn't that sudden after all. I had been ignoring the gentle nudges (i.e. symptoms) that something (inflammation) was festering in my body for many years. Some of the early warning signs seemed "normal." After all, I am not alone in thinking that everyone has skin issues, headaches, muscle aches, joint pain, ulcers, and fatigue. We have come to accept that "common" means normal.

But wait, there's more. During this most challenging time, my almost four-year old son was diagnosed with Pervasive Developmental Disorder (an autism spectrum disorder). Like me, he too had shown some early "warning signs"—his heart rate was dropping in utero (which resulted in an induction at 36 weeks), he had body tremors in the first days of life, jaundice, difficulty nursing (inability to latch); he went on to miss all his developmental milestones, like walking, rolling over, crawling, babbling, pointing. He had chronic gas pain and bloating. He had sensory issues and colic. At the age of two and still non-verbal, we began Early Intervention and by the time he was four years old, but prior to the autism diagnosis, he had multiple diagnostic labels including speech disorder, apraxia of the body and mouth, sensory processing disorder, selective mutism, panic disorder, anxiety, and significant cognitive delays (slow processing speed).

I have come to believe that I was following a path that was not meant for me and something drastic needed to change. It's fascinating how the universe works to make sure you receive your lessons loud and clear.

And the lesson didn't stop there. My mother, a young 71-year-old, has cerebellum ataxia, a degenerative nerve issue in the part of the brain that controls muscle coordination. Ironically her degeneration was detected at the same time of my physical breakdown and my son's diagnosis, but I never knew. It took seven years before her body gave up the fight and she began falling down. Her leg muscles were not responding to physical therapy. She had a car accident but didn't "know" it and soon began to speak with slurred speech. She was having difficulty forming her thoughts and getting her words out. And then she had a grand mal seizure! Her window of opportunity to reverse this degeneration in her brain had passed. This felt unacceptable! I often wonder what her life would be like today if more doctors where trained to understand the role that nutrition plays in preventing chronic and degenerative disease.

Each one of our stories demonstrates the wisdom of the body. All of these conditions, although different in presentation and severity, share the same hidden connection—an immune response to something in our environment. Our food.

We were all having an immune response to otherwise healthy food. We were triggering an inflammatory process in our body leading to a cascade of symptoms that when added up presented as a debilitating disease. We were unknowingly feeding our disease. As you will learn throughout this book, I will explore the various factors that play into many chronic conditions of the body.

We've all heard about the power of good food in the diet, but what may surprise you (as it did me), is the degree to which nutrition plays a role in preventing and healing many chronic conditions including seemingly unrelated symptoms like bloating, diarrhea, reflux, mood swings, anxiety, chronic fatigue and so much more. It's true—many of these symptoms and conditions stem from nutritional deficiency and/or reactions to certain foods we consume every day.

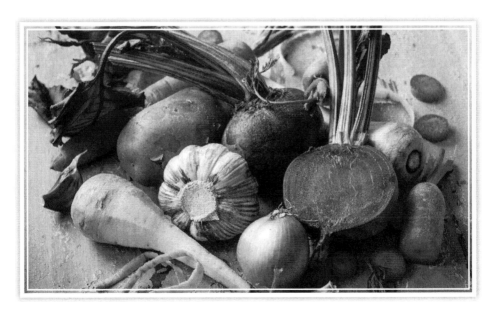

When I first suspected nutrition might have an impact on my disease and brought up a food connection to my treating physicians I was met with discouragement over and over. And as any stubborn, redhead, Irish girl would do, I decided to explore it on my own. I became more and more intrigued (and angry). There was a connection.

Why aren't people getting accurate information about nutrition and its role in disease treatment and prevention? The science is there to support the benefits of nutrition in reversing many, if not all, chronic conditions. I decided to take a deeper look into the published research and the evidence-based reports on the effect of nutrition on all systems of the body—particularly, digestive, endocrine, neurological, and muscular. I became fascinated with the immune system and our microbiome—our inner eco-system. I was not only committed to learning about issues that I struggled with but those that affected my family and that commonly affect many people in my own community. So, I wrote this book and founded an organization called Rhode to Health to help inspire people to seek accurate information and to prompt a curiously around health that leads to wellness and vitality at all stages of life.

Have you ever wondered what messages your body is sending you?

Writing this book caused me to reflect back on this time in my life when I faced the same questions. I felt frustrated and alone. I took on the task of exploring my own illness when I reached the end of the line with ineffective treatments for my own diseases.

What if your joint pain, fatigue and/or mood swings was caused by something you were doing? Maybe you received a diagnosis from your doctor that only describes your set of symptoms but offers little solutions. If you don't know what's causing or triggering your condition, then you can't reverse it. Medications are simply masking the underlying root case of illness and dysfunction.

The Hidden Connection is for you if you are interested in the answers to your own questions around health. It's an opportunity to step back from the volume of conflicting information around nutrition and health and get back to the basics. What is your body telling you? It's for people who want to be proactive in finding solutions to their health complaints and for healthy people who want to avoid developing chronic disease and autoimmune conditions that are preventable when you recognize the early warning signs as the wisdom of the body.

I want to change the way people perceive chronic disease. I believe the human body has the innate power to heal itself if given the support and opportunity to do so.

We must start by lifting the **burden** off the body.

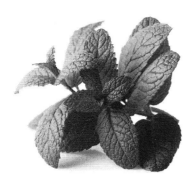

What to expect from this book:

The Hidden Connection will help you to uncover the clues behind your day-to-day ailments and your on-going health concerns. This book does not address every dis-ease or symptom in the body nor it is intended to provide a detailed protocol for healing. Instead it focuses on helping you to uncover the early warning signs of dis-ease and how to use food as medicine when you are faced with chronic conditions.

It is also important to understand my use of the word disease. When I use the term disease I am referring to *dis-* meaning "without" and *ease*. In this book disease re-fers to a condition a person experiences, including sickness, illness, discomfort, or a disorder that produces symptoms.

I will share personal stories of dis-ease from my own family that will help you discov-er the potential disorders lurking in your own home and, more importantly, inspire you to take control of your health once and for all. I know you are busy. I intentional-ly simplified the concepts in this book so you could get through it quickly and start healing today. I know it will change your life.

Guaranteed!

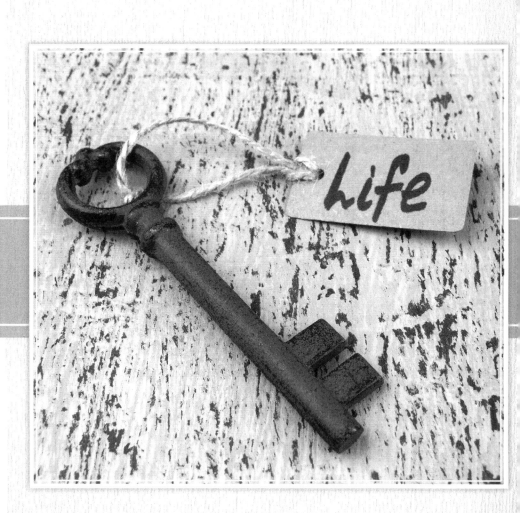

THE D.E.A.P.™ APPROACH

I created the **D.E.A.P.** approach to wellness to take you through the four basic steps of transformation: *Discovery, Education, Action, and Prevention.* I believe one of the biggest obstacles keeping people from achieving their wellness goals is feeling overwhelmed by the process and the fear of change.

The notions of sacrifice, discomfort and inconvenience permeate the mind when people think of resolving their health issues. The word "diet" is always associated with deprivation. Interestingly, the word diet actually means "the course of life; the way of thinking or living."

The D.E.A.P. approach became the roadmap to my way of living. It delivered a sense of liberation I had never felt around food or health. My mind shifted from deprivation to deliberation. I felt informed, connected to my body and more in control of my health outcomes. I was empowered. I stopped measuring the quality of my health by the size of my jeans. It can do the same for you. Here is the breakdown of the transformational process:

Discovery

What are your symptoms really telling you? Discover what your body is telling you in the form of symptoms. If you don't identify the wisdom of the body as early warning signs you'll miss the opportunity for a healthy life.

Everything you need to know is happening everyday in the form of symptoms like constipation, yeast infections, acne, chronic pain, migraines, arthritis, memory loss, mood swings, fatigue, asthma, anxiety, depression, loss of libido, weight loss resistance, and more.

Instead of consistently suppressing it with medications, numbing it with alcohol, masking it with caffeine and in many cases feeding it with sugar, you can use it as powerful information to uncover the root of your most nagging health complaints. When you continue to ignore or even learn to accept the symptoms as "normal," the root cause continues to persist. We are then left with chronic inflammation in the body—which becomes disease!

Education

Once you recognize, or discover, the symptoms as abnormal and reversible, you can begin to understand why they exist. Learning the foods and lifestyle choices that are contributing to a dis-eased state is the next (and most important) phase of healing. I believe one of the primary reasons people fall back into old patterns is because they never received the education needed to maintain health.

Understanding the function of the human body is critical. I'll use digestion as an example: The digestive system is the center of the immune system. Nutritional deficiencies can result from poor digestion and poor assimilation of the nutrients. Our digestive system is the home of hundreds of different species of bacteria that influence our health. Certain foods can trigger the release of specific hormones in the digestive system that can influence our risk for certain diseases.

All systems—digestive, neurological, endocrine, respiratory, cardiovascular, circulatory—function together in an interconnected way. You must always treat the whole body (the person) not the individual parts. You are whole.

In addition to the function of the body, there are so many areas that require education like environmental triggers, exercise, detoxification, energy, sleep, food combining, metabolism, bacteria, and other internal stressors. But without addressing the whole body, one is still chasing symptoms. Education is key. Finding a practitioner or health coach that is willing to teach you is an important step in maintaining health and wellness.

Action

Here is where the magic happens. Turning your knowledge into action by rebuilding the gut and digestive system as the foundation for health. A strong immune system requires proper digestion and a healthy gut. Our inner eco-system, also known as our microbiome, is our vitality. Whether you're dealing with chronic disease, weight issues, learning disorders, or chronic pain, you must improve the health of your gut. Our microbiome was treasured by our ancestors but goes largely ignored today. It is the place to initiate all forms of healing.

In fact, what you eat has a huge effect on you, your family, and the people in your life. However, what you absorb in your intestines when you eat is even more important. The best diet in the world will leave you disappointed if you lack the ability to absorb nutrients in the gut on a daily basis.

Removing foods that are triggering your immune system and creating internal inflammation throughout your body is critical. Your intestinal mucosa is constantly regenerating and repairing itself. However, you can't expect your body to heal when it's under constant assault. This is essentially what's happening when you consume foods that your body is sensitive to.

There are so many things you can do from your own kitchen that can support healing, vitality and long-term wellness. Getting back to the basic and traditional practices of food preparation can have long lasting effects on your health.

Prevention

Once you have the tools, you can manage your health instead of managing disease. You'll know when to stop and listen to the early warning signs (symptoms!) and take action to address the issue at the root level before it becomes chronic. Learning to navigate the world of food in social settings and marketing mayhem is critical to long-term success. You become aware of your role in maintaining a healthy body and mind.

By using your body as your guide, you remain in the driver's seat of your own health. I encourage you to learn about your body and talk to your doctor about your concerns as an expert in your own physiology. Going to the doctor's office as if it's a repair shop will result in test after test to search for clues only to hear a list of diseases you don't have or a "label" that describes the symptoms you already knew.

Self-care is the most effective form of disease prevention. It bridges the gap between you and the healthcare system. It gives you the control over your own health outcomes. Self-care starts with nourishing food and exercise but goes beyond diet and addresses relaxation, setting boundaries, moments of joy, and exploring what makes you feel "alive."

Practices like relaxation, mindfulness, and yoga can prevent chronic stress from damaging your health. Setting boundaries around things that are important to you, like taking time for yourself, reminds others that you value your needs too. Forgetting to nurture yourself puts you at risk for unhappiness, feelings of resentment, and burnout. You can be a better caretaker for others when you are well. In a sense, self-care is good for you and everyone else.

Turning back to Mother Nature as a guide can nourish your mind, body, and spirit. When you eat seasonally and locally, your body is more in tune with the natural order of things and able to maintain balance from the inside out. Instinctively, your body craves seasonal foods, like cooling, raw foods in the summer and grounding root vegetable in the fall and winter to add warmth. Sabotaging this natural rhythm by eating processed foods that hijack your taste buds and internal messages is what holds you back.

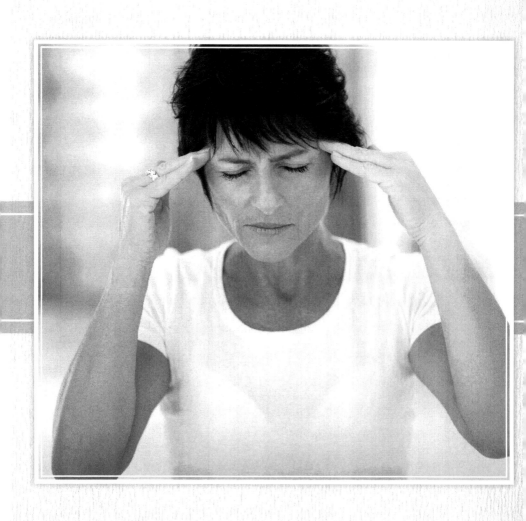

Part I: Discovery

Wisdom of the Body

Symptoms as your teacher

Millions of people, just like you, are struggling with the viscous cycle of chronic symptoms that are associated with internal inflammation and immune dysregulation. For a long time, scientists have linked arthritis, edema, and irritable bowel syndrome (IBS) to inflammation, but only recently have we been able to make the connection to diabetes, certain cancers, and other degenerative diseases. Even heart disease, once thought to be caused by high cholesterol, is now linked to various forms of inflammation.[1]

Inflammation plays an important role in fighting infections. When we catch a cold or virus, our body responds appropriately by elevating body temperature in the form of a fever to fight back or a runny nose or cough to clear mucous. These symptoms are expressions of the inflammatory process. There are also other reasons for internal inflammation like broken bones, bruises, cuts, parasites, fungal infections, and more. Ideally, when the job is done, inflammation goes away. But what happens when the inflammatory process does not go away? We are left with chronic inflammation.

Any disease ending in *"itis"* refers to an inflammatory condition, for example arthritis, bronchitis, or colitis. Any tissue, cell, or organ in the body can be affected. Acute inflammation or the kind you expect with pain, swelling, and redness, is usually short-lived and gone in a matter of days. Chronic inflammation is another story. This kind of inflammatory condition can linger for years.

While chronic inflammation is a common thread in all disease, determining the root cause of inflammation can be challenging. The truth is no one thing will determine whether you develop a chronic disease or an autoimmune disorder. You simply can't look at the body in isolation from its environment. Our environment, including food, chemicals, emotions, and behaviors, influences our genes to create a state of health or in some cases a state of dis-ease.

Understanding this relationship between environment and genes is called *epigenetics* and understanding it is the foundation of the functional nutrition model. Epigenetics is the study of changes in gene expression caused by certain base pairs in DNA or RNA being "turned off" or "turned on" again, through chemical reactions.[2]

In terms of understanding chronic disease, many practitioners will describe epigenetics in this way "the genes load the gun, the environment pulls the trigger." Environment refers to the air, water, food, exercise, toxins, chemicals, and emotions we are exposed to daily. It was once believed that our chances of developing disease were predominantly related to our genes with little focus on the environment. We now know that the opposite is true. A study, published by the American Journal of Human Genetics, reveals how human genes interact with their environment to boost disease risk. You have more control over your health than you think. This is great news!

THE BODY DOESN'T LIE

Functional nutrition, in particular, looks at the systems of the body and uses symptoms to identify imbalances. The symptoms are signals from the body that something is not functioning as it should be. To understand the impact of environment on our health, we turn to symptoms to provide the clues. When the physical body is functioning properly, you are able to digest foods (without bloating, gas, and pain), assimilate nutrients from your food (without supplementation), eliminate waste and toxins (without enemas, laxatives, and heavy detox programs), sleep and recover (without medication and suppressants). You can essentially stop "managing" symptoms.

When it comes to nutrition, always consider your individuality rather than the 'one size fits all' diet. More often than not, people attempt to fit into a dietary theory rather than discover a dietary approach that is right for them. One of the best lessons I learned came from the Institute for Integrative Nutrition (IIN) where I was taught "how to think," not "what to think."

It's a program that teaches more than one hundred dietary theories offering each student the opportunity to explore their own unique dietary requirements. Experimentation with foods was encouraged and it was the beginning of my own awareness that there was no such thing as the perfect diet. There was however a diet that was perfect for me, and that's where my attention needed to go. Discovering how food was affecting my health was key. I later went on to explore the role of functional nutrition, which differs from the conventional approach most notably by addressing root cause to illness and nutritional deficiencies linked to many conditions.

I applied this approach to myself and my oldest son who was diagnosed with Pervasive Developmental Disorder—not otherwise specified (PDD-nos), an autism spectrum disorder.

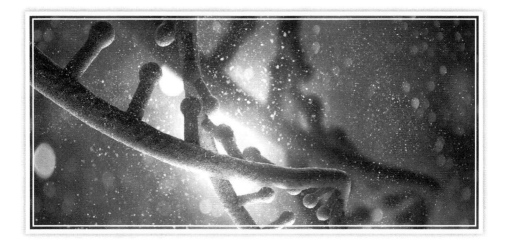

We started with a gluten-free diet and saw some improvement. I knew we needed to keep exploring. Autism is a complex disorder with many different causes. We approached Stephen's health issues from all angles. The key is to recognize chronic symptoms as clues. As I attempted to understand autism in an effort to help my son, I found very little information about nutrition. Instead, I observed a system where millions of dollars are spent on the research into genetics (we had no family history of autism) and the brain (I viewed my son's struggle as a whole body disorder). So, when I shifted my attention away from this thinking (genetics and brain) and applied the functional nutrition approach, we started seeing measurable results. I discovered the inflammation in his brain was coming from inflammation in his gut (the second brain).

Now, let's explore what chronic symptoms may look like for you and how they relate to internal inflammation, imbalances, and poor functioning. I will also discuss what might be at the root of the problem and why medications and/or supplements are not always the best solution (and in many cases, may be making matters worse.)

Of course, everyone wants relief from their symptoms. However, the symptoms are feedback from the body and when we remove them without getting to the root cause, we prevent our body from healing. For example, if you take a pain reliever medication for a headache, the symptom will disappear but the cause of the headache may still be manifesting in the body leading to internal inflammation and compromised health. Discovering what's "triggering" the headache is critical.

Another common chronic symptom that people struggle with is heartburn. People often describe their heartburn, acid reflux or gastroesphageal reflux disease (GERD) as "too much" stomach acid. They believe the stomach acid is overflowing, causing it to flow upward into the esophagus. The truth is, this is really a case of too little stomach acid or poor functioning of the esophageal sphincter, the ring of muscles at the lower end of the esophagus. When it's functioning properly, the sphincter relaxes to allow food to pass through to the stomach, but otherwise it remains closed. According to Dr. Marc Rothenberg of Cincinnati Children's Hospital Medical Center, when people were treated for asthma, the condition of the esophagus improved. He believes that there is a connection between food, environmental allergies, and the esophagitis.

Here's what we know. The sphincter stays closed when the proper amount of stomach acid keeps it closed—in essence there is a natural "pressure" within the stomach. When our stomach acid drops too low, this sphincter relaxes, allowing acid to travel into the esophagus causing pain and irritation. So, in this example we can see that treating the symptom can lead to even greater problems because the conventional treatment would be to "suppress" stomach acid even more, making you more vulnerable to bacterial overgrowth and other issues associated with low stomach acid. The acid is there for a reason. We need it to break down our foods properly and protect our body from pathogens. Low stomach acid leads to a cascade of health issues, which I will cover more in part II of this book under the digestive system.

I suffered for years, starting at the age of sixteen, with a duodenal ulcer. I received prolonged treatment including prescription acid suppressors because of the false belief that I was producing too much stomach acid. I was fortunate to find a forward-thinking doctor at the time, who recognized the connection between the Helicobacter Pylori infection (H. Pylori) and treated me with antibiotics. Research supports that removing this bacteria often results in the healing of ulcers, which it did for me. However, there's a twist. Some scientists believe that this bacteria is there for a reason and that altering our microbiome by removing the H. Pylori bacteria, we may be setting up long-term health consequences we don't fully understand. Unfortunately most people, today are still being prescribed stomach acid suppressants for the treatment of ulcers and heartburn which can lead to parasitic or bacterial infections that your stomach acid would normally destroy. Once these organisms arrive in the small intestines, they can thrive and create a whole host of health problems.

In fact, when it comes to chronic conditions, many people start off with mild symptoms like constipation, diarrhea, and bloating, which they describe as "normal for me." They have digestive issues, which later become Irritable Bowel Syndrome (IBS). Their history of headaches becomes chronic joint pain or hormone imbalances. Then, the weight loss resistance kicks in followed by an autoimmune diagnosis and a list of prescription medications that don't appear to be working.

HERE ARE COMMON SYMPTOMS (OR DISORDERS) OFTEN ASSOCIATED WITH THE SAME ROOT CAUSE:

- Digestive issues: bloating, gas, constipation, diarrhea, IBS

- Sleep issue, chronic fatigue, insomnia or waking throughout the night

- Asthma, congestion, sneezing, or coughing

- Muscle aches, joint pain, or arthritis

- Dark circles under your eyes

- Dull hair and/or brittle nails

- Skin issues, including acne, rosacea or eczema

- Mood problems, like aggression, mood swings, depression, anxiety, irritability

- Weight gain or weight loss resistance

- Autism, ADD or ADHD

- Colitis, Crohn's disease

- Asthma or shortness of breath

- Brain fog, fuzzy thinking, lack of focus

- Canker sores in mouth

- Headaches, including migraines

- Infertility

- Fibromyalgia

- Hashimoto's or thyroid issues

- Depression, anxiety

What could be at the root of these problems? Surprisingly, it's intestinal hyper-permeability or "leaky gut," along with other (often co-existing) conditions like gut dysbiosis (bacteria imbalance), candida, low stomach acid, small intestinal bacterial overgrowth (SIBO) and food sensitivities.

Leaky gut is often overlooked or ignored by the medical profession, especially in the absence of digestive symptoms. And, in most cases there are no digestive complaints. Once the body develops leaky gut, the likelihood of developing food allergies and sensitivities appears inevitable. This starts the cascade of health-related problems that affect all parts of the body and even our emotional health.

THE ROOT OF ALL DISEASE BEGINS IN THE GUT

> *"All disease begins in the gut"*
> ~ Hippocrates

The gut is the place to start healing—not cure disease. Research has linked leaky gut to many health concerns and seemingly unrelated chronic diseases.[3]

With more people affected by chronic stress, toxic overload, inflammatory diets, and bacterial imbalance in the gut, the prevalence of leaky gut and gut related issues, like candida overgrowth and small intestinal bacterial overgrowth (SIBO), is becoming epidemic.

Like your exterior skin, the intestinal lining serves as an inside barrier between the outside environment (food, drink, bacteria) and the internal environment (blood stream and organs). In order for the gut to absorb nutrients from our food, there is some permeability. Think of the lining as a piece of fine mesh cloth protecting your body and blood stream from anything harmful but flexible enough to absorb small molecules. However, when the lining is damaged or hyper-permeable, meaning the tight junctures of the intestines are loose or damaged, this creates an opportunity for harmful parasites, bacteria, toxins, undigested food particles, and more to enter the blood stream where they don't belong. This condition results in an immune response by the body.

A mucosal barrier covers the lining of the gastrointestinal tract, from the mouth to the anus. It provides your immune defense against pathogens (infectious agents) as well as the proper processing of food antigens (substances that prompt antibodies causing an immune response). The mucosal barrier is also present in the sinuses, genital and urinary tracts, among other areas. The mucosal barrier contains specific immune defenses (antibodies) known as sIgA, IgA, IgG and IgM. This is why allergy lab testing must look beyond IgE-antibody testing.

In the case of leaky gut, one or more of the antibodies for dietary proteins, yeast, aerobic bacteria and/or anaerobic bacteria, is elevated. This means the mucosal barrier is damaged and proteins (antigens) are entering the general circulation (where they don't belong). Unless you support your gut to allow the mucosal barrier to repair, the body will remain in a chronic inflammatory state as the immune system is triggered and fighting back.

This is the beginning of the battle between food and body. It's when nourishment turns to systemic inflammation. It's the beginning of the chronic symptoms and, if left untreated, will lead to autoimmunity. It's where you must START your journey back to health.

SO WHAT DAMAGES THE GUT IN THE FIRST PLACE? POSSIBLE CAUSES INCLUDE:

- Antibiotics or medication (including steroidal or non-steroidal) that decrease or disturb the normal gastrointestinal flora and damage the gut lining. Common NSAIDs include: Advil / Motrin (ibuprofen), aspirin, Aleve /Naprosyn (naproxen sodium).

- Dysbiosis (or gut flora imbalance) caused by candida, parasites, infections, or fungi. This means you have more "bad" bacteria than "good". You want the good bacteria to be dominant.

- Repetitive consumption of processed foods and/or inflammatory oils.

- Genetic manipulation of foods and/or pesticides/herbicides added to our foods like glyphosate, found in genetically modified foods (GMO)

- Poor digestion due to low stomach acid production and/or enzyme deficiency.

- Unrecognized food sensitivities or allergens like gluten, soy, or casein in the diet.

- Food additives, dyes, and preservatives in the diet.

- Chronic stress—physical or emotional—due to decreased immune function or adrenal fatigue as a result of chronically elevated cortisol.

- Alcohol, drug, and medication abuse.

- Premature weaning of infants to solid foods. Often foods that are difficult to digest (like grains) are introduced to babies when the gastrointestinal tract is not fully developed. Baby formula and cow's milk can also be difficult to digest.

- Environmental toxins—metals, chemicals, pollutants, or pesticides—can disrupt gastrointestinal flora.

Throughout this book I will review many of the common contributors to a damaged gut in more detail and give you the basic understanding of how they happen and what you can do about it.

Well fed, but undernourished

As far back as ancient Greek and Roman times, vitamin and mineral deficiency were recognized and treated as diseases. More recently, scientists are discovering the important role that vitamins and minerals play in the function of the human body. They are powerful substances that perform many tasks to maintain health and vitality and a deficiency can present as a variety of symptoms, many of which should be addressed by a qualified healthcare practitioner.

Deficiencies in vitamins and minerals can also inhibit your body's natural ability to heal. A diet comprised mainly of processed foods is automatically void of vitamins and minerals. Processed food is also guilty of chelating, or binding, existing vitamins and minerals from the tissue in your body. Beyond this issue, consider how nutrient deficiencies ties back to poor gut health. If the gut is damaged, its ability to absorb nutrients is compromised.

You absorb your nutrients in the gut, particularly the small intestine, so if the gut is unable to do this important job, it leaves you vulnerable. Some of the most shocking signs of gut dysfunction for my mother were present during childhood. At the age of fifteen, her teeth fell out requiring a full set of dentures (sorry mom). Imagine this for one moment. Why on earth would a young girl be losing her teeth? And more importantly why didn't anyone ask the bigger question of what was at the root of her problem? Of course I was not alive nor was I privy to any conversation between my grandparents and the dentist. However, I can tell you that my mother has no idea why it happened and diet was never explored. What comes to mind for me immediately is poor nutrient absorption in the gut. Oral health is strongly linked to gut health.

When it comes to issues of oral health, I turn the pioneering work of Dr. Weston A. Price, DDS. Dr. Price traveled the world in the 1930's to study the oral health and bone structure of thousands of people in various primitive populations (tribes) in order to understand how nutrition affected health. His research determined that traditional diets produce better physical health and emotional stability than diets based on convenient, modern foods. These traditional diets provided nutrient levels that far exceed the minimum requirements for adequate nutrition. His findings, which can be found in his book *Nutrition and Physical Degeneration* (originally published in 1939), are still relevant today. These findings clearly show that dental cavities and deformed dental arches, resulting in crowded, crooked teeth and unattractive appearance, are a sign of physical degeneration, resulting from nutritional deficiencies.

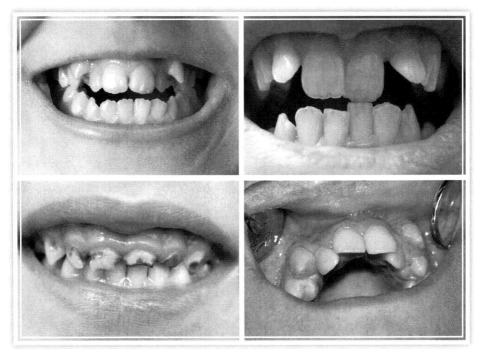

"A variety of dental issues commonly seen in children today; Dr. Weston A. Price's research indicates that these conditions are in fact not genetic but, instead, caused by a lack of vital nutrients during the formative period of the body."

Micronutrient deficiencies can also be diagnosed with blood tests, which you can request at your annual physical. Unfortunately the solution isn't as easy as popping a supplement for whatever you are lacking or taking a multi-vitamin. Often times the nutrient you are deficient in is a reflection of another nutrient that is out of balance. The same is true for excess amounts. A good example of this is too much iodine. Often people with thyroid autoimmune conditions have excess iodine but this can be due to selenium deficiency. When selenium levels are corrected, the iodine levels are brought back to normal.

I believe supplementation should be used only as needed and that micronutrients should be obtained through whole food as much as possible. Again, the more effective way to counter poor absorption is to address the root cause by healing in the gut. Doing otherwise is actually chasing external solutions to an internal problem. Once gut health has been restored, you can then explore other reasons for deficiencies.

When our son, Stephen, was diagnosed, and even earlier when he showed multiple developmental delays, it seemed obvious to me that he was out of balance (literally and figuratively). Research tells us that children diagnosed with autism spectrum disorders, ADHD, and developmental delays experience a higher rate of vitamin and mineral deficiency.[4]

The nutrients most commonly deficient include vitamins, minerals, essential fatty acids, digestive enzymes and amino acids.

HERE ARE JUST SOME OF THE KEY NUTRIENTS WE USED TO ADDRESS STEPHEN'S DEFICIENCIES:

- Essential Fatty Acids

- B vitamins—especially B6 and B12

- Magnesium

- Zinc

- Vitamins A, C, D, E and K

Evaluating an individual child's nutrient deficiencies can lead to dramatic shifts in development. The benefits he experienced from nutrient therapy were improved eye contact, decrease in self-stimulating behavior (arm flapping, joint compression, jumping to regulate himself), improved language, and improved social and cognitive function.

Autism spectrum disorders, including ADHD, are complicated conditions in which nutritional and environmental factors play major roles. Larger studies are needed to determine optimum multifactorial treatment plans involving nutrition and environmental changes in addition to effective behavioral, education, speech and physical therapies. However, there is so much we do know about the role of diet and nutrient deficiencies and I believe we are obligated to start there.

I can still remember sitting in the waiting room at the hospital and therapy clinics waiting for Stephen's occupational or physical therapy session to begin. The room was filled with children with special health care needs eating donuts and blue slushy drinks with stressed out parents doing their best to get through the day. I couldn't help but wonder the impact that those foods were having on these children. How would they manage to get through the therapeutic exercises and occupational tasks like learning to write, lacing their shoes or riding a bike, which already came with such difficulty? At the time, I didn't know just how much food impacted the body and mind, but intuitively I knew what they were eating was working against their goals of getting the most from their therapy session.

Minerals: The Fabulous Four

Here is additional information on several micronutrients and how a deficiency can present major health problems.

Calcium

You know calcium is important for your bones and teeth. But do you know it plays an important role in muscle contraction, blood pressure, blood coagulation, energy production, immune system function, nerve conduction, and brain function?[5]

Calcium regulates the speed, intensity, and clarity of every message that passes between neurons and signals the uptake and release of neurotransmitters. Calcium also interacts with potassium and sodium to maintain proper levels of nerve-cell stimulation, which balances nerve cell activation and inactivation on the brain. Calcium also interacts with zinc in the regulation of histamine (a neurotransmitter) and is dependent on DHA (a fatty acid that is commonly low in children on the spectrum) for all membrane functions.[6]

The most commonly consumed foods in America today include sugar, soda, and processed foods, which are highly acidic. Many experts believe these foods force the body to leach calcium from the natural supply in our bones and tissue. This is the body's attempt to neutralize the acid leaving us vulnerable to abnormal bone formation and poor bone strength.

Bone formation is a complex process with many micronutrients. Calcium is the principle mineral working together with phosphorous. When these nutrients are not absorbed in sufficient amounts, weak or deformed bones can result. This is another reason to address the health of the gut where nutrient absorption takes place as well as reduce the processed foods that deplete minerals from the body. Deficiency of calcium not only leads to poor dental health but also soft bones and osteoporosis, if left untreated.

Those with dairy sensitivities (common for children on the spectrum and women) are at risk for low calcium intake. Supplementing with non-dairy food sources such as leafy greens, almonds (almond milk and almond butter), sunflower seeds, sesame seeds (sesame butter/tahini), beans, blackstrap molasses, lamb, carob, figs, and broccoli is important. For children who refuse to eat these foods, one solution is to grind them down and hide them in other foods like meatballs or in smoothies.

Supplemental calcium is tricky, as it requires magnesium and vitamins D and K for optimal absorption. Calcium carbonate is not very absorbable while calcium citrate or calcium malate are preferred. I do not suggest calcium aspartate because some people may have trouble with the aspartate as it can have neurotoxic effects similar to glutamate (MSG).

The recommended daily intake of calcium is 800–1200 mg from a combination of food and supplement sources. For kids up to 8 years of age, 800 mg is recommended.

Calcium-rich foods

- Broccoli (Raab), 1 bunch   500 mg

- Collards, 1 cup   245 mg

- Kale, 2 cups   200 mg

- Almonds (dried), 2 oz   148 mg

- Sesame seeds, 1 Tbsp   88 mg

Note: Vitamin D is responsible for calcium and phosphorus metabolism related to bone and tooth formation and regulates the body's absorption of calcium. Magnesium also helps protect your bone health.

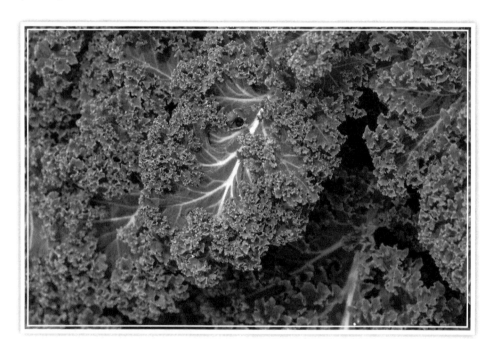

Magnesium is needed for more than three hundred biochemical reactions in the body. It helps maintain normal muscle and nerve function, keeps heart rhythm steady, supports a healthy immune system, and makes our bones strong. Magnesium also helps regulate blood sugar levels, promotes normal blood pressure, and is known to be involved in energy metabolism and protein synthesis.[7,8] There is an increased interest in the role of magnesium in preventing and managing disorders such as hypertension, cardiovascular disease, and diabetes. Dietary magnesium is absorbed in the small intestines and is excreted through the kidneys.

Magnesium's benefits can include reduced symptoms of chronic pain, fatigue, and insomnia. Magnesium may also provide protection from a number of chronic diseases, especially those associated with aging and stress.

Magnesium is known to reduce muscle tension, lessen pain associated with migraine headaches, improve sleep, and address neurological disorders such as anxiety and depression. Low levels have been linked to fibromyalgia, ADD, and restless leg syndrome and more.

So much of my medical treatments included painkillers, antibiotics and cortisone that all deplete the body of magnesium. In addition, my chronic inflammation, surgery, poor gut health and hormone imbalances were conditions that required an increased amount of magnesium. I had so much pain and stiffness that there were days that I honestly felt like the tin man; Magnesium was my "oil can." It still is.

It wasn't until 1990 that the American College of Rheumatology established diagnostic criteria for fibromyalgia. While this provided the official "label" for the illness, it offers little understanding of the condition and no treatments.

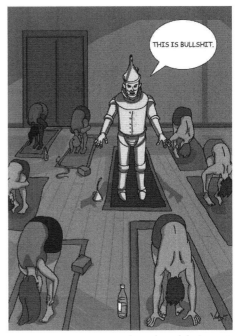

Image by vashdesigns.com

Fibro means "connective tissue" and *myalgia* means "muscle pain." Dr. Carolyn Dean, author of *The Magnesium Miracle*, believes fibromyalgia is an accumulation of toxins and infections of the environment. So in addition to relaxing muscles and transporting energy, magnesium is also used as a master detoxifier.

MAGNESIUM-RICH FOODS:

- Pumpkin seeds, 2 oz   300 mg

- Spinach (cooked), 1 cup   156 mg (raw spinach, 24 mg)

- Lentils, 1 cup   148 mg

- Mackerel, 3 oz   82 mg

- Avocado   56 mg

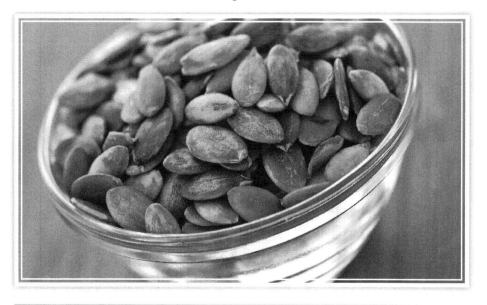

ZINC

Zinc is an essential mineral that is naturally present in some foods and available as a dietary supplement. You may be familiar with Zinc as a common ingredient in cold lozenges and over-the-counter cold remedies.

Zinc is involved in numerous aspects of cellular metabolism. It is required for the catalytic activity of approximately one hundred enzymes and it plays a role in immune function, protein synthesis, wound healing, DNA synthesis, and cell division. Zinc also supports normal growth and development during pregnancy, childhood, and adolescence and is required for proper sense of taste and smell. The body has no specialized zinc storage capacity so daily intake is required to maintain optimal amounts.[9]

In children, a zinc deficiency can present as irritability and tearfulness. Deficiency can lead to gaze aversion, susceptibility to infection and inflammation, poor wound healing (including leaky gut), and eczema.[10]

Common warning sign of zinc deficiency include poor taste and smell, white lines in fingernails, loss of appetite, or compromised immune system.

It is worth noting that copper and zinc work together, so it is important to have sufficient copper. However, copper is not normally the element that is in deficiency.

THE ZINC CHALLENGE

You can test if you need zinc with a taste test. If it tastes sweet, pleasant, or like water, then your body needs it. If it has a strong metallic or unpleasant taste, you are not zinc-deficient and there is no need to supplement.

How do to the Zinc Taste test

Take two teaspoons of liquid zinc sulphate (I recommend Designs by Health Zinc Challenge) and hold it in your mouth for ten to thirty seconds.

ONE OF THE FOLLOWING CATEGORIES SHOULD BE APPLICABLE TO YOUR RESPONSE OF TASTING TWO TEASPOONS OF THIS SOLUTION:

- No specific taste while holding the solution in your mouth indicates a very low zinc level.

- A slight taste, resembling hydrogen peroxide, indicates a low zinc level.

- An immediate, strong, metallic taste indicates adequate zinc levels.

- The sooner and stronger the taste of this product is noticed, the more zinc is present in the body.

Usage: If you fall into the first two categories take 1 to 4 tablespoons per day until a strong metallic taste is noticed.

Selenium is a trace mineral and antioxidant. Selenium deficiency is often found in those with digestive health issues such as Crohn's or celiac disease, or those with serious inflammation due to chronic infection.[11] Selenium deficiency may not cause illness by itself, but instead makes the body more susceptible to illnesses caused by other infections due to its role in immune function.

A deficiency in selenium is commonly linked to those with thyroid issues, including Hashimotos, making selenium a critical element in protecting the thyroid gland from damage and balancing the body's iodine levels.

Selenium can be toxic in excess, so I recommend dietary supplementation in the form of two raw Brazil nuts per day to meet the recommended dosage of 100 to 200 mcg/day.[12] Other sources of selenium (although not has high as Brazil nuts) include, crimini mushrooms, cod, shrimp, tuna, halibut, salmon, scallops, chicken, eggs, shiitake mushrooms, lamb, and turkey.

VITAMINS

Vitamin deficiency is associated with chronic disease. According the Journal of American Medical Association, vitamin deficiency syndromes are less common today, however, suboptimal intake of some vitamins is a risk factor for chronic diseases and common in the general population. Suboptimal folic acid levels, along with suboptimal levels of vitamins B6 and B12, are a risk factor for cardiovascular disease, neural tube defects, and colon and breast cancer. Low levels of vitamin D contribute to osteopenia and fractures; and low levels of the antioxidant vitamins (vitamins A, E, and C) may increase risk for several chronic diseases.

Sadly, most people do not consume an optimal amount of all vitamins by diet alone leaving them vulnerable to chronic disease.

WATER-SOLUBLE VITAMINS:

Deficiencies in water-soluble vitamins are less likely to lead to chronic disease and autoimmune disease compared to fat-soluble vitamins (A, D, E and K), however they still play an important role in managing overall health and indirectly modulating the immune system.

Vitamin C

When vitamin C is insufficient in the body, you can begin to experience rough skin, poor wound healing, and bleeding gums. Vitamin C is responsible for the synthesis of collagen, a principal component of skin tissue. It is an antioxidant with anti-inflammatory properties and supports immune function by controlling the damage caused by oxidants or free radicals.

B-Complex Vitamins:

THERE ARE EIGHT B VITAMINS AND THEY ALL PLAY AN IMPORTANT ROLE IN CELLULAR METABOLISM. THEY ARE:

- Thiamine (B1)
- Riboflavin (B2)
- Niacin (B3)
- Pantothenic Acid (B5)
- Pyridoxine (B6)
- Folate (B9)
- Cobalamin (B12)
- Biotin

B vitamins break down carbohydrates into glucose, which provide energy for the body. They break down fats and proteins, which aid the functioning of the nervous system. They support muscle tone in the stomach and intestinal track as well as the health of our skin, hair, eyes, mouth, and liver.

According to the Linus Pauling Institute, other nutrients depend on B vitamins to metabolize properly, for example vitamin B6 is required to convert tryptophan (an amino acid found in protein) into Niacin (B3). Classic niacin deficiency causes a condition called pellagra, the symptoms of which include dermatitis, dementia, and diarrhea. If left untreated, the condition can lead to death.

In addition to restoring tissue health, B vitamins promote and maintain healthy skin including the prevention of rosacea, eczema and dermatitis. They also support proper immune system function by reserving the body's antibodies, which guard against infections, as well as, protecting the nervous system. Low levels of vitamin B6, folate and vitamin B12 also lead to poor formation of red blood cells.

People with conditions consistent with B vitamin deficiency, despite a diet including foods rich is B vitamins, may want to consider the health of the gut and poor absorption as the potential link to chronic symptoms. People eating a vegan or vegetarian diet need to supplement with a high-quality B Complex vitamin.

I'm not sure we will ever escape the "low fat" diet craze. Time and time again, people claim to eat a healthy diet but continue to avoid good dietary fats. A diet deficient in fat becomes a diet deficient in fat-soluble vitamins. While research has proven the false claims that saturated fat causes cardiovascular disease, misinformation continues to circulate in the medical field and in our society.[13]

The most common mistake is the use of processed seed oils like canola, corn, soy and margarine in place of saturated fats like butter, lard, tallow, olive oil and coconut oil. Besides the fact that the seed oils are genetically-modified, they are high in omega-6 polyunsaturated fats which are inflammatory. Imitation butters are also full of trans fats that raise your LDL (low) cholesterol while lowering your HDL (good) cholesterol.

All the fat–soluble vitamins, which we get from high quality animal products (which means cows grazing on grass not in confinement eating soy and corn under artificial light), have the potential to regulate the immune system. Many believe one of the reasons autoimmune diseases are on the rise is the result of our shift away from animal fats including butter, tallow, and lard from grass-fed animals.

Deficiencies in vitamins A, D, and E have been linked to a variety of autoimmune conditions. Fat-soluble vitamins work synergistically as a team. Vitamins A and D tells cells to make certain proteins; after the cellular enzymes make these proteins they are activated by vitamin K.

One of the simplest ways to consume adequate levels of fat-soluble vitamins A, D and K is by supplementing with a blend of butter oil and fermented cod liver oil by Green Pastures (available online). This eliminates the risk of an overdose in one.

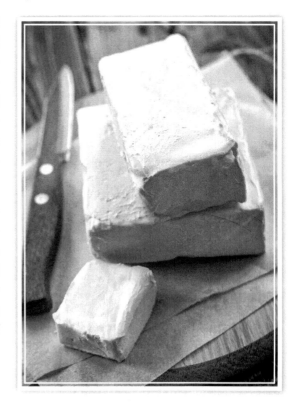

Part 1: Discovery Takeaways

Everything you need to uncover the hidden connection
to your health issue is happening everyday
in the form of symptoms.

Functional nutrition looks at the systems of the body
and uses symptoms to identify imbalances.

The body doesn't lie.

Inflammation in the brain can come
from inflammation in the gut.

The gut is the place where you must start any healing process.

Leaky gut is largely under diagnosed and is linked to many health
concerns and seemingly unrelated chronic diseases.

Deficiencies in vitamins and minerals can inhibit
your body's ability to heal and thrive.

When you ignore or accept symptoms as "normal,"
the root cause continues to persist.
Medication is a band-aid, not a solution.

You don't have to have all the answers to start the discovery
process. You just need the courage to take the first step.

Ask yourself today:

What is my body telling me?

Am I making excuses about my symptoms?

Am I eating nutrient-dense foods every day?

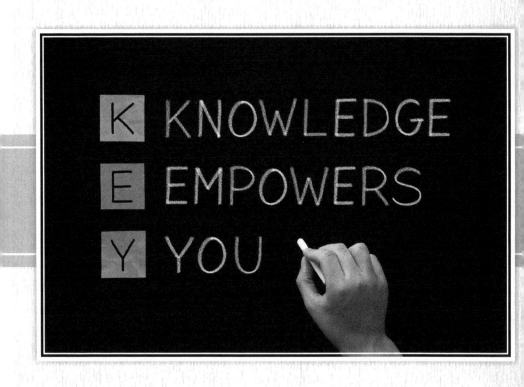

Part II: Education

Learning the Basics to Avoid the Pitfalls

DIGESTION 101 AND COMMON DIGESTIVE DISORDERS

In order to understand the impact of what's happening inside your body you must first break down the function of the digestive system and some of the common reasons why you may be missing the key to unlock your health issues.

Poor digestion is very common these days and tummy complaints are not always present for those with poor digestive function. What sets this dysfunction in motion can be as simple as our behaviors around eating. We no longer prioritize the time and energy needed to digest our food. We often eat on the go, we wait too long between meals, and then we eat at a frantic pace. We rarely honor our need to "rest and digest."

We also have little understanding of proper food combining and often eat foods together that require different digestive speed and enzymes. A good example of this is the summer cookout when we grill up hamburgers and then eat watermelon for dessert without taking in to account that meat takes up to three hours to digest and melon takes about twenty minutes. So, eating the melon after the meat is a digestive nightmare often resulting in bloating, digestion distress, and gas. Not exactly what you had in mind for a day at the lake. Like many fruits, melons make a great snack, and are best eaten alone.

PRE-DIGESTION: WHERE IT ALL BEGINS

What you eat is important, but what you digest is even more important. The most complicated foods for the body to digest are carbohydrates. Carbohydrates include grains, beans, vegetables, fruits, nuts, seeds, sugar, starches, herbs, and spices. Carbohydrate digestion starts in the mouth when we chew our food. Each food group—carbohydrates, proteins, and fats—require different enzymes to break down the food and support the digestive process.

- Amylase is secreted from the parotid glands and breaks down carbohydrates.

- Protease is secreted from the submandibular glands and begins protein digestion.

- Lipase is secreted from the sublingual (under the tongue) glands to initiate fat digestion.

The importance of chewing in the digestive process is often overlooked. Chewing is necessary to expose as much surface area as possible on the food particles so that enzymes can begin digestion. If the food is not chewed thoroughly, this puts a stress on the digestive system especially if there is any digestive difficulty.

People with chronic illness or poor digestion (these often go hand in hand) should chew their food until it is almost liquid (which will feel impossible). This takes stress off the body and can do much to help repair the digestive tract. One of the reasons the *GAPS* diet, created and presented by Dr. Natasha Campbell-McBride in her book *Gut and Psychology Syndrome,* is so successful with autoimmune disease is the emphasis on "pre-digesting" the food by cooking or blending all the meals.

After swallowing, the food moves through the pharynx and esophagus, which make up the pathway to the stomach. When food enters the upper part of the stomach, it begins to expand the stomach. The lower part of the stomach remains flat and closed while the upper part opens to accommodate the food. During the time that the food sits in the upper section, acid secretion in the stomach is minimal for at least thirty to forty minutes.

Digestive enzymes from the saliva and in the food itself are still at work. The more digestion that happens here, the less work the body has to do later.

THE ROLE OF DIGESTIVE ENZYMES

My first introduction to the benefits of digestive enzymes was a book by Dr. Howard Loomis called *Enzymes: The Keys to Health.* I was so fascinated by his observations around the functions of digestive enzymes some of which seemed to describe the missing puzzle pieces for my ongoing issues. He wrote, "Most people who acquire symptoms of musculoskeletal dysfunction, such as osteoporosis, herniated discs, bursitis, and leg cramps, do not readily digest protein."[14] I had all of these symptoms and had been told by a surgeon that I needed steel rods in my back due to aggressive facet joint degeneration, an opinion I thankfully disagreed with. Loomis suggests that the body's ability to digest and assimilate protein would consequently improve

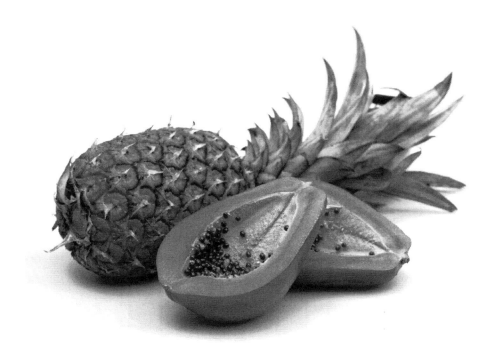

its ability to carry calcium and other minerals to the tissues. While we know much more about the role of digestive enzymes today, I was intrigued by his early observations and the connection between digestion and illness. I wanted to know more.

I have come to view digestive enzymes as the "construction workers of the body." The human body provides a fair amount of different enzymes for digestion, mostly from the pancreas and cells lining the gut wall. Within the small intestine the enzymes derive nutrition from food then use the vitamins and minerals as building materials to maintain the body.

As a certified raw food chef, I often get questions about the benefits of raw foods verses cooked. Is one better than the other? And the short answer is: they are both important. The right choice for you would depend on the condition of your health and your overall goal.

While raw food is naturally full of enzymes, vegetables are covered in a thin coating of cellulose. Human do not manufacture cellulose, the enzymes needed to break down this type of fiber, and must rely on the fermentation by the flora in the large intestine. According to Devin Houston, Ph.D. and enzyme biochemist at Houston Enzymes, "The enzymes present in raw foods exists only in amounts sufficient to degrade the food over a period of several days." He further explains, "Since digestion occurs within hours, not days, the actual contributions of food enzymes towards digestion is minimal."

A popular comment among veggie lovers is the notably strong bodies of cow's that survive eating grass. Of course the reason for this is due to the cow's ruminary stomach that is divided into four chambers and can hold massive amounts of cellulose-digesting microbes to break down the grass and hay that make up such a large part of its diet. This is why they can get big and strong from eating grass.

This does not mean raw foods are not beneficial for you if you have health issues. Instead, the health of your digestive system should be considered when you are addressing your nutritional needs. In fact, your diet should change to meet the needs of your current state of health. For those eating a primarily raw food diet, keep in mind that enzymes can be supplemented. I suggest a brand that uses a concentrated form by fermentation of certain non-pathogenic fungi. The enzymes are then purified from the fungi through many biochemical procedures leaving an enzyme concentration significantly higher than what's found naturally in raw foods.

People with autoimmune disorders, including autism, often have gut damage. This was certainly the case for our son Stephen. His lack of digestive enzymes caused by an inflamed and leaky gut was a major contributor to his long list of symptoms. In additional to correcting some of the nutrient deficiencies, reducing yeast overgrowth, and regulating his bowel movements, the digestive enzymes provided additional support during and after his gut healing protocol when it came time to reintroduce certain foods.

Another symptom that concerned us was his "addiction behavior" around certain foods like bread and cheese, a common complaint among parents raising kids with autism. Gluten and casein are the proteins found in these foods and are noted for producing exorphin peptides (opioid-peptides) after contact with pepsin and elastase enzymes during digestion. I can still remember the look in his eyes when the bread basket was delivered at restaurant meals. If you, or your child, acts "addicted" to certain foods, a 30-day elimination of these foods is always worth exploring.

The gluten-free/casein-free diet was our first line of defense. We knew the offending foods had to go. You'll learn more about this important step in section III. After listening to a lecture by Dr. Houston on the promising benefits of specific peptidase enzymes called dipeptidyl peptidase IV, or DPP IV, which degrades exorphin peptides, we decided to experiment with the reintroduction of high-quality raw dairy from grass-

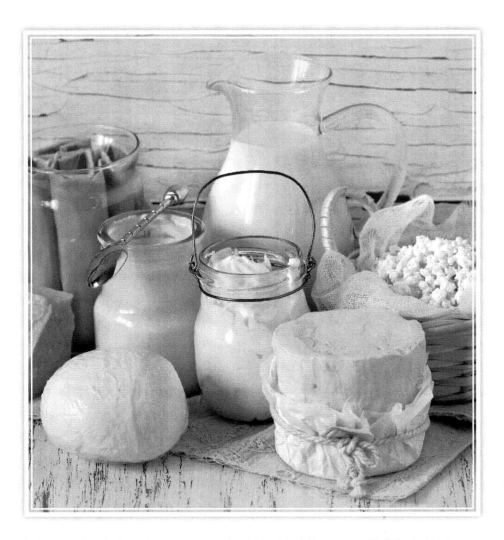

fed cows. If and when dairy is re-introduced, it should be raw and full-fat (whole)—not pasteurized or lactose-free industrial dairy products.

The benefits of using digestive enzymes are worth considering. After all we all want improved nutrient absorption from our food and better digestion. Studies have determined the safety of digestive enzymes with no toxicity or adverse side effects, even when taken in extremely large doses.[15, 16, 17, 18, 19] Dosage is based on meal size and not the weight or age of individual. Ideally, enzymes should be taken at the beginning of each meal to increase contact time with food in the stomach. For young children, the capsules can be opened and sprinkled on the food or can be purchased in a chewable form.

THE ROLE OF THE STOMACH

The stomach is our powerhouse with a high concentration of hydrochloric acid. The stomach creates the acidic environment needed to digest protein and ionize minerals. This is why is it common for vegetarians to experience heartburn or reflux, due to lower consumption of dietary protein and therefore a natural decrease in stomach acid. People who switch between diets can also experience symptoms of low stomach acid, which they don't realize can improve on its own as the body adapts or by supplementing with hydrochloric acid to aid in the digestion of proteins. The proper function of hydrochloric acid in the stomach for digestion is key to prevent the risk of anemia, thyroid problems, osteoporosis, and autoimmunity.[20]

You want the goldilocks amount of stomach acid. Just the right amount of stomach acid is key. Too much stomach acid is known as hyperchlorhydria, which is rather rare. Most people have too little. In addition to the digestion of food in the stomach, the hydrochloric acid also plays a role in stimulating the release of bile from the gallbladder to effectively metabolize fat in the small intestine. So, when people are experiencing gallbladder "issues," the first place they may want to look is the stomach, to rule out low stomach acid.

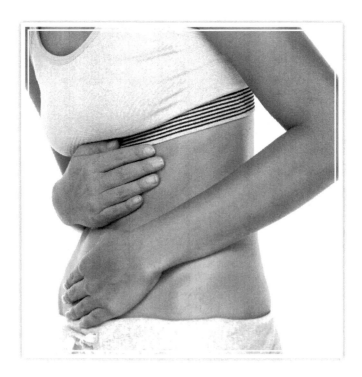

Low stomach acid in a very common problem especially in older individuals or those who have suffered from various infections like *H. Pylori*, or those who have been on antibiotics and other medications like non-steroidal anti-inflammatories. Low stomach acid sets the stage for damage to the delicate lining of the digestive tract and the formation of leaky gut syndrome.

SYMPTOMS ASSOCIATED
WITH LOW STOMACH ACID

- Bloating, belching, heartburn, or gas
- Diarrhea or constipation
- Chronic fatigue or adrenal fatigue
- Dry skin/dandruff
- Rectal itching or candida
- Multiple food allergies and/or sensitivities
- Weak, peeling or cracked fingernails

POSSIBLE CAUSES
OF LOW STOMACH ACID:

- Poor diet, excess sugar, or processed foods
- Mineral or vitamin deficiencies
- Chronic infections
- Use of antibiotics
- Age (we produce less stomach acid as we age)
- Use of acid blocking medications
- Use of NSAID (Tylenol, aspirin, ibuprofen)
- Use of birth control pills
- Chronic stress

Fortunately, there are many natural ways to stimulate an increase in stomach acid production, including the use of digestive bitters, supplementing with betaine HCL, peppermint tea after meals, and spices that promote digestion.

Digestive bitters, which are liquid herbal formulas, help to support the stomach acid production and have been used for centuries to aid in the digestive process. Another simple remedy is to drink a cup of strong peppermint tea after meals. This is often sufficient to reduce excess gas production. Many common spices also have gas-relieving properties and offer digestive support, such as cardamom, caraway, anise, and fennel. In Indian restaurants, for example, it is typical to chew a handful of raw anise seeds after a meal to aid digestion.

Commonly used bitter herbs also include ginger root, peppermint leaf, and cayenne pepper. These herbs or spices can be found at your local natural food market.

Lastly, taking digestive enzymes will help to more thoroughly break down and digest food. Often due to stress, pharmaceuticals, or existing gut inflammation we produce inadequate amounts of these enzymes.

Supplementing with Betaine HCL

Pepsin is naturally produced in the stomach when there is enough stomach acid. Individuals with low stomach acid will not be able to produce the active form of this vital protein-digesting enzyme. To improve stomach acid production and protein digestion, it is best to supplement with betaine HCL and the proteolytic enzyme pepsin. This is available over the counter at any health food store. A word of caution for anyone with a history of ulcers; always check with your health care practitioner as HCL supplementation can irritate ulcers.

Risks of low stomach acid

When you have low stomach acid you are unable to effectively break down protein in the stomach. This allows very large proteins to get into the small intestine and creates major stress on the pancreas to produce enough enzymes to metabolize the proteins.

This ultimately creates stress and irritation throughout the gut. It also leads to insufficient absorption and utilization of key amino acids that make up the protein molecules. Incomplete digestion can lead to leaky gut syndrome and trigger autoimmune activity in different regions of the body. Also, improper digestion may lead to small intestinal bacterial overgrowth (SIBO), candida overgrowth, and other parasites. It also creates an acidic blood stream and depletes minerals throughout the body. Mineral depletion leads to the inability to form stomach acid and the vicious cycle continues.

Sadly, the current medical approach to treating low stomach acid, which presents as heartburn and GERD, continues to be the use of acid stopping drugs. Unfortunately, these drugs not only bypass the underlying cause of these problems, but may make it worse. So people who start taking antacid drugs end up taking them for the rest of their lives. This is a serious problem.

Acid stopping drugs promote bacterial overgrowth, weaken our resistance to infection, reduce absorption of essential nutrients, and increase the likelihood of developing IBS, other digestive disorders, and even cancer. The manufacturers of these drugs are aware of these problems. When acid-stopping drugs were first introduced, it was recommended that they not be taken for more than six weeks. Clearly this advice has been discarded, as most people are on these drugs much longer. It is estimated that drug companies make more than $7 billion a year selling these medications.

For more information on the role of stomach acid and conditions related to inefficient amounts, I recommend the book, *Why Stomach Acid is Good for You* by Jonathan Wright, M.D.

THE INTESTINES

The intestines are where most absorption of nutrients and water takes place. It's a long, continuous tube running from the stomach to the anus. The intestines include the small intestine, large intestine, and rectum. The not-so-small intestine is about twenty feet long and gets its name because it is about an inch in diameter. Its job is to absorb most of the nutrients from our diet. Mucosal tissue lines the small intestine, which is divided into the duodenum (first part), jejunum (middle and primary site of nutrient absorption), and ileum (final part that empties into the large intestine).

Microscopic examination of the mucosa tissue reveals that the mucosal cells are organized into finger-like projections known as villi with each square inch of mucosa containing around 20,000 villi. The cells on the surface of the mucosa also contain finger-like projections of their cell membranes known as microvilli, which further increase the surface area of the small intestine. It is estimated that there are around 130 billion microvilli per square inch in the mucosa of the small intestine. Wow!

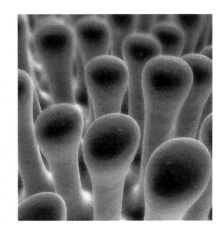

Once nutrients are absorbed by the villi, they are transported throughout your body via the bloodstream. The mucosal wall of the intestine is considered semipermeable, which means the pores allow certain things to enter the bloodstream while blocking others. For instance, nutrients are allowed to pass through but toxins and large undigested food particles are blocked.

When a person has celiac disease, it is the villi that become damaged when the person eats the dietary protein gluten. They become flat and unable to absorb nutrients from food leaving the individual deficient is essential nutrients for life. Visualize a plush shag carpet that becomes a flat, industrial indoor-outdoor carpet. That's villi atrophy.

In the case of leaky gut, the problems begin when the wall of the small intestine is damaged. Food particles and toxins that should be blocked pass through the small intestine triggering the immune system to attack. The problem is the immune system doesn't just build up antibodies to the food particles; it attacks your healthy cells, too. This is one of the ways food allergies lead to autoimmune disorders.

It takes nearly twenty-four to thirty hours to complete digestion with most of the work happening in the small intestine. The large intestine (colon) completes the process. At about five feet long and about three inches in diameter, the colon's main job is to absorb water from waste, creating stool. As stool enters the rectum, nerves there create the urge to defecate.

The large intestine is full of friendly bacteria called commensal bacteria that help in absorption of vitamins made by the bacteria. There are over 700 species of bacteria that perform a variety of functions in the large intestine.

These bacteria produce large amounts of vitamins, including vitamins A, K and the B vitamins. When your vitamin intake in your diet is low, this can be an important source of these vitamins. A person who depends on absorption of vitamins formed by bacteria in the large intestine may become vitamin deficient if treated with drugs like antibiotics that kill the commensal bacteria.

The large intestine plays an important role in immunity. The lymphatic tissues of the large intestine help in the production of antibodies and cross-reactive antibodies. These antibodies are produced by the immune system against the normal commensal bacteria but may also be active against related harmful bacteria and thus prevent infections.

One of the most common disorders of the large intestine is constipation. Most health care practitioners label constipation when you experience on three or fewer bowel movements a week. From a functional standpoint, lack of a daily bowel movement is considered constipation and should not be overlooked as a sign of dysfunction. Remember digestion is completed in twenty-four hours, so if you are going days without eliminating waste from you intestines, your health and your mood will suffer. Irritation is one of the biggest side effects to poor elimination, as well as, feeling or acting "uptight."

Common causes of constipation include inactive lifestyle, too much processed foods, lack of hydration, lack of dietary fiber and of course as you now know low bacteria count in the colon. Changes in routine can also trigger digestive stress and lead to constipation, especially at times of travel when access to bathrooms is an issue or decrease activity level.

Keep in mind that constipation is also a common side effect of medications, including but not limited to antacids, diuretics, narcotics and antidepressants. Americans spend more than $600 million a year treating constipation and over the counter laxatives can be very habit forming and lead to further digestive stress.

COMMON DIGESTIVE DISORDERS

SMALL INTESTINAL BACTERIAL OVERGROWTH (SIBO)

Have you ever had a flat stomach upon waking in the morning but by dinnertime you look like you're in your second trimester of pregnancy? Even if you haven't experienced this extreme version of abdominal swelling, any amount of bloating is not normal. It is a symptom of intestinal inflammation. If gas and bloating is a regular part of your day, small intestinal bacterial overgrowth (SIBO) could be to blame.

SIBO is a condition in which the amount of bacteria in the small intestine is too high. The small intestine is a sterile environment and bacteria from the large intestine (your colon) can relocate to the small intestine where is does not belong. There are two potential reasons for this to happen; For some it is a decrease in migrating motor complex, which is the process that moves bacteria down in the large intestine after clearing it from the small intestine after digestion; and for others, it is a physical obstructions like damage from Crohn's disease or diverticulitis that can cause an abnormal buildup of bacteria in the small intestine instead of passing it on to the colon where it belongs. It then feeds off foods in your diet, namely carbohydrates and sugar, causing the bacteria to multiply and "overgrow."

Diets high in sugar, refined carbohydrates, and alcohol can also negatively influence the health of the gut and the bacteria. And of course, medication that disrupt the normal bacteria, such as antibiotics, steroids, and acid blocking drugs, are also to blame.

I can still remember being told that "passing gas is not normal" at an appointment with a naturopathic doctor when my son was diagnosed with autism. Honestly, I thought the woman was nuts. My initial reaction was, everyone has gas (which is true). However, frequent or excessive gas is "common" but not "normal" and it's a classic sign that the health of your gut needs attention. She was right. I just wasn't ready to admit there was a problem. When the student is open, the lesson will be learned.

DISORDERS LINKED TO SIBO

SIBO has consequences beyond gas and bloating (that's just your red flag). Here's what you really need to consider. Bacterial overgrowth damages the lining of the small intestine, resulting in poor digestion, poor nutrient absorption, and inflammation. SIBO has been associated with many conditions, including but not limited to, the following:

- Scleroderma
- Diverticulosis
- Diabetes
- Crohn's disease
- Celiac disease
- Rosacea

- Restless leg syndrome
- Fibromyalgia
- Parkinson's disease
- Hypothyroidism
- Rheumatoid arthritis

HOW DO YOU KNOW IF YOU HAVE IT?

Testing methods vary among practitioners and labs. One method is a fasted lactulose or glucose breath test done over a three-hour period either in a practitioner's office or using a take-home kit. The test requires a one-to-two-day preparatory diet, a baseline breath sample, and drinking a sugar solution of either glucose or lactulose. The diet removes the common food that would normally feed the bacteria as to allow a clear reaction to the sugar drink solution. Once the baseline is established, the 3-hour testing period begins with samples collected at designated intervals by exhaling your breath through a thin tube.

Many practitioners prefer the lactulose breath test over a glucose test because lactulose can travel to the lower part of the small intestine, whereas glucose does not. Two types of exhaled gas are tested: hydrogen and methane. These two gases are produced only by bacteria, not humans. Hydrogen is associated more with diarrhea, while methane has been shown to be associated with constipation. Knowing which type of gas is released by SIBO would dictate the appropriate treatment.

Once SIBO has been detected there are a number of things you can do. Although I have an aversion to antibiotics given their overuse and the potential harmful side effects, it is important to recognize that they have their place in certain situations.

The antibiotic, rifaximin (prescription required), has a ninety-one percent success rate for treating SIBO. One advantage to this choice is rifaximin does not travel outside the intestines and does not cause candida (yeast overgrowth), which is a common complaint with antibiotic use. When methane gas is present, the antibiotic neomycin may be added (in addition to rifaximin), for better results.

Herbal antibiotics, including garlic extract, berberine, oregano oil, and cinnamon have reports of success as a treatment option, although they have been less studied.

The diet commonly used to address SIBO is the Specific Carbohydrate Diet (SCD), which limits specific sugars, called disaccharides (two sugar molecules) and starches, called polysaccharides. The SCD diet and the science behind it was made popular by Elaine Gottschall in her book "Breaking the Vicious Cycle." It is based on the principle that some people, like those with SIBO, cannot digest carbohydrates due to damage in the small intestine. The bacterial overgrowth present with SIBO then feeds off the sugar of the disaccharides.

For those with SBIO the SCD diet is often used in combination with the fruits and vegetables indicated in the low FODMAP diet.

THE ACRONYM **FODMAP** STANDS FOR:

> **F**ermentable
>
> **O**ligo-saccharides (Fructans and Galacto-oligosaccharides (GOS))
>
> **D**i-saccharides (Lactose)
>
> **M**ono-saccharides (excess Fructose)
>
> **a**nd
>
> **P**olyols (Sorbitol, Mannitol, Maltitol, Xylitol and Isomalt)

FODMAPs are foods that are poorly absorbed in the intestine, which means they can be left there to ferment and therefore cause the symptoms of IBS. When too many sugars enter the intestine they can feed bacteria which leads to a production of excess gas. A FODMAP intolerance can lead to bacterial overgrowth. So for those with SIBO eating foods high in FODMAPs can exacerbate symptoms.

A low FODMAPs diets is appropriate for anyone suffering from gastrointestinal issues. Too often people rely on a quick-fix (i.e. medication) without addressing the diet and that is a recipe for disaster.

Examples of food sources for each of the FODMAPs are listed below. For a complete list of high and low FODMAP foods see page 39. I recommend that you consult with a nutrition practitioner who is experienced with a low FODMAP diet.

- FRUCTANS: Artichokes, garlic (in large amounts), leeks, onion, onion powder, shallots, wheat (in large amounts), rye (in large amounts), barley (in large amounts), inulin;

- GALACTO-OLIGOSACCHARIDES (GOS): Legume beans (baked beans, kidney beans), lentils, chickpeas

- LACTOSE: Milk, icecream, custard, dairy desserts, condensed and evaporated milk, milk powder, yoghurt, soft cheeses (ricotta, cottage, cream, mascarpone).

- EXCESS FRUCTOSE: Honey, apples, mango, pear, watermelon, high fructose corn syrup;

- POLYOLS: Apples, apricots, avocado, cherries, nectarines, pears, plums, prunes, mushrooms, sorbitol, mannitol, xylitol, maltitol, and isomalt.

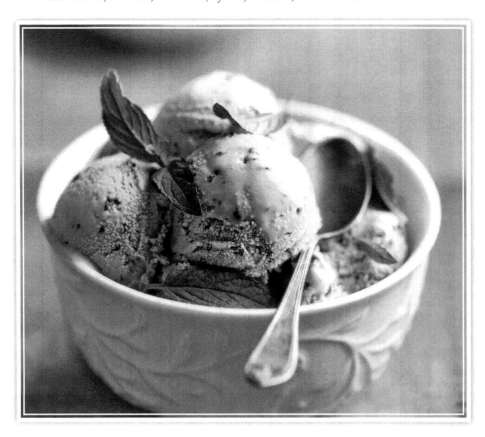

FODMAPs Foods[21]

CAUTION: HIGH FODMAPs	
Lactose	Milk, evaporated milk, yogurt, ice cream, custard, and certain cheeses such as ricotta, cottage, and mascarpone
Fructose	Fruits such as apples, pears, peaches, mangoes, and watermelon; coconut milk; coconut cream; dried fruits; and fruit juices
	Sweeteners such as agave and honey
	HFCS-based products such as BBQ sauce, ketchup, and pancake syrup
	Alcohol such as sherry and port wine
	Sodas with HFCS
Fructans	Vegetables such as artichokes, asparagus, Brussels sprouts, broccoli, beetroot, cabbage, chicory, garlic, leeks, okra, onions, radicchio lettuce, shallots, and snow peas
	Grains such as wheat and rye
	Added fiber such as inulin and fructo-oligosaccharides; watch items such as probiotic supplements, granola bars, and frozen desserts
	Fruits such as watermelon
Galactans	Chickpeas, lentils, kidney beans, and soy products
	Vegetables such as broccoli
Polyols	Fruits such as apples, apricots, blackberries, cherries, nectarines, pears, peaches, plums, prunes, and watermelon
	Vegetables such as cauliflower, button mushrooms, and snow peas
	Sweeteners such as sorbitol, mannitol, xylitol, maltitol, and isomalt (sugar-free gums/mints, cough medicines/drops)

SAFE: Low FODMAPs	
Lactose	Lactose-free versions of milk, cottage cheese, ice cream, and sorbet; certain cheeses such as cheddar, Swiss, Parmesan, and mozzarella
Fructose	Fruits such as ripe bananas, blueberries, grapefruit, grapes, honeydew, lemons, limes, passion fruit, raspberries, strawberries, and tangelos. Sweeteners such as sugar and maple syrup
Fructans	Vegetables such as bok choy, bean sprouts, bell peppers, butter lettuce, carrots, celery, chives, corn, eggplant, green beans, tomatoes, potatoes, and spinach
	Garlic-infused oil
	Gluten-free* breads/cereals, rice and corn pasta, rice cakes, and potato and tortilla chips
Galactans	
Polyols	Fruits such as bananas, blueberries, grapefruit, grapes, honeydew, kiwi, lemons, limes, oranges, passion fruit, and raspberries
	Sweeteners such as sugar, glucose, and aspartame

CANDIDA (CANDIDA ALBICANS)

Candida overgrowth is another common disorder of the intestines. It is a fungal organism (yeast) that exists naturally in the body, in small amounts. Most people associate candida with vaginal infections in women or thrush in babies. Surprisingly, candida can be very helpful, as it aids in digestion and nutrient absorption. However, it can grow out of control and cause a whole lot of health problems like:

- Fatigue
- Brain fog
- Sugar cravings
- Allergies (food or seasonal)
- Digestive issues
- Anxiety or depression
- Skin rashes

Overgrowth of candida happens when the bacteria in our gut becomes compromised or unbalanced. Ideally, our gut contains more than one hundred trillion cells of "good" bacteria, which keeps candida in check. Chronic stress, antibiotics, birth control pills, poor diet and other lifestyle factors can easily upset this delicate balance, creating an environment where candida can thrive. And like a bad house guest, candida can be tough to get rid of.

Candida overgrowth creates a vicious cycle in the body. Foods that help candida thrive like sugar—in any form (glucose, fructose, sucrose)—are standard in the American diet. Normally, a strong immune system and healthy gut can keep yeast under control. However, when yeast does overgrow, they release a toxic by-product called acetaldehyde. Acetaldehyde produces symptoms of an alcohol hangover. Sometimes you can experience "giddiness" from yeast that presents as silliness in kids or inappropriate laughter in adults.

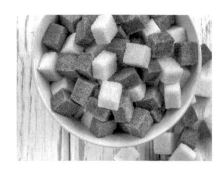

In addition to the symptoms I mentioned above, other possible signs of candida overgrowth include, skin and nail infections like athletes foot, ringworm and toenail fungus, feeling tired, skin issues like eczema, psoriasis, rashes and hives, rectal itching, strong carbohydrate cravings, mood swings and irritability, and seasonal allergies or itchy ears.

Candida is very common with kids on the autism spectrum. My son definitely showed signs of candida overgrowth. Even today he is sensitive to sugar, including healthy forms like fruits. If his candida begins to overgrow, he develops a red ring around his upper lip. Visualize severely chapped lips. Now that we know the cause we can quickly bring him back into balance by adjusting his diet (removing sugar) and increasing his probiotics. We also make sure he is getting enough rest and we apply essential oils for topical relief.

One of the best diets and approaches to treating candidiasis is The Body Ecology Diet by Donna Gates. In her book, she includes a questionnaire developed by Dr. William Crook, which is fairly accurate for self-diagnosis of candida.

According to Donna, candida can grow in your blood, where it becomes a systemic infection. The yeast thrive on your dietary nutrients (minerals, proteins, and fats) which leads to further deficiencies especially for minerals (iron, selenium and zinc). Interestingly, these minerals are commonly deficient in people with autoimmune.

Fortunately, the intestines are constantly regenerating, and you always have the opportunity to turn things around. In Part III of this book, I will review the steps to building the foundation of health including the four basic steps to gut healing: **Remove** (irritants), **Replenish** (digestive power), **Repair** (mucosal barrier) and **Restore** (good bacteria) along with traditional foods/practices that support healing and nourish the body from the inside out.

TEST YOUR TRANSIT TIME

A HEALTHY TRANSIT TIME IS 18 TO 24 HOURS.

1. Swallow a handful of white sesame seeds following your "test" meal. Note the date and time of this meal.

2. Watch your bowel movements over the course of the next few days for the seeds. You will be looking for largest amount not just a few scattered seeds. They will be intact.

3. Note their "arrival" time.

If the seeds arrive fast (less than 18 hours) you may be eating foods that irritate your digestive system. If the seeds arrive late (after 24 hours) you should work to improve your digestion. Things to consider would include dietary fiber, the health of your gut flora (probiotics), proper hydration, and the benefits of digestive enzymes.

Hormones 101 and common endocrine disorders

A Brief Introduction to the Endocrine System

Hormones are not just for teenagers or for women during that "time of the month." Everyone has hormones and they have a larger impact on your body than you realize. The endocrine, immune and nervous systems are interconnected therefore health conditions affecting one system will impact the others often leading to symptoms in various areas of the body.

The endocrine system, also called the hormone system, consists of many glands, such as **thyroid, pancreas, thymus, gonads (ovaries and testies), adrenals, para-thyroids,** and the controlling **pituitary pineal** and **hypothalamus glands**. They make up a complex system and communicate by sending messages to each other through the release of hormones into the bloodstream. The hypothalamus sends a special hormone-encoded message to the pituitary gland giving it instructions, and the pituitary gland then manages all the other glands. The hypothalamus is a bit like the chief executive, with the pituitary the managing director over all the other glands. Once the message hits a receptor cell, it gives the cell instructions that get carried out from creating energy from sugar to triggering ovulation.

The messages sent are responsible for controlling and regulating many body functions such as metabolism, growth, body temperature, sleep, menstruation, ovulation, labor, menopause, and many other functions.

The complex hormonal changes within a woman's body are often antagonistic which means that life changes like pregnancy or menopause can often trigger the beginning or worsening of a hidden chronic illness. It's not uncommon for women to report "things have never been the same since my pregnancy."

When one gland is over or underactive, the other glands feel the effects and suffer as well. This hormone imbalance can also occur if the liver or kidneys are not working properly as their function is also important for clearing hormones from the blood.

Why do I want you to understand the endocrine system? Everything is connected. You must take the time to understand how your body works if you want to understand how it might be working against you.

HYPOTHALAMUS

The hypothalamus is a portion of the brain that links the nervous system to the endocrine system via the pituitary gland. It stimulates certain hormones that in turn stimulate or inhibit the hormones secreted from the pituitary gland.

The hypothalamus is also responsible for the messages controlling body temperature, sleep, fluid and electrolyte balance, levels of adrenalin, metabolism and blood pressure. It basically sends endocrine signals to the pituitary gland.

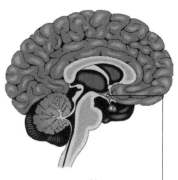

HYPOTHALAMUS

THE PITUITARY GLAND

The pituitary gland is located at the base of the brain. It is attached to the hypothalamus and no larger than a pea. It is the "master gland" of the body, influencing the rest of the functions of the endocrine glands in the body. Imagine something that small having so much power in the body! The pituitary gland is divided into three sections, or lobes, and each one produces different hormones, which then act in certain ways to send messages to other parts of the body.

The **anterior lobe** is responsible for the production of growth hormones:

- PROLACTIN: Stimulates the production of breast milk shortly after delivery;

- ADRENOCORTICOTROPIC HORMONE (ACTH): Stimulates the adrenal glands;

- THYROID STIMULATING HORMONE (TSH): Stimulates the thyroid gland

- FOLLICLE STIMULATING HORMONE (FSH) AND LUTEINIZING HORMONE (LH): Stimulate the ovaries in women and testes in men.

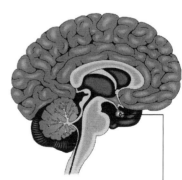

THE PITUITARY GLAND

The **intermediate lobe** produces melanocyte-stimulating hormone, which controls skin pigmentation. Finally, something to blame for the freckles!

The **posterior lobe** produces antidiuretic hormone (ADH), which increases the absorption of water into the blood by the kidneys.

PINEAL GLAND

The pineal gland is fascinating to me. It is located deep in the brain above and behind the pituitary gland, and produces melatonin through the synthesis of serotonin, a hormone responsible for the control of sleep patterns. It is about the size of a grain of rice.

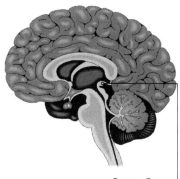

PINEAL GLAND

Often called the **"third eye,"** it is considered our internal antenna or our connection to higher consciousness. It responds to light through messages from the retina, hence its ability to regulate sleep patterns and biological functions. Melatonin is secreted in response to the length of darkness making the pineal gland a central part of developing our circadian rhythm. With today's modern conveniences of light and technology, we stay stimulated much later into the night, which alters this natural circadian rhythm.

Consequences of prolonged circadian disruption lead to reduced melatonin and a variety of cancers. Melatonin suppression due to prolonged exposure to light at night among female nurses has been associated with an increased risk of breast and colorectal cancer.[22] Male night-shift workers have been found to have an increased risk of prostate cancer.[23]

Patients with rheumatoid arthritis have disturbances in the hypothalamic-pituitary-adrenal (HPA) axis. These are reflected in altered circadian rhythm of circulating serum cortisol, melatonin and interleukin-6 (IL-6) levels and in chronic fatigue.[24]

The thyroid gland is located in the neck close to the windpipe. It consists of two lateral lobes joined by the isthmus, which is a small piece of tissue and is a butterfly shape. It produces two hormones, which control metabolism, T3 (triiodothyronine) and T4 (thyroxine). T4 is also converted into T3 in the cells and tissues of our body. If too much is secreted then the body works in overdrive with symptoms such as diarrhea, rapid heart rate, otherwise known as hyperthyroidism. Likewise if too little is secreted, as in hypothyroidism, the body becomes sluggish and you will have a tendency toward things like constipation and weight gain.

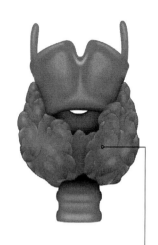

THYROID GLAND

The control center behind the thyroid is the **pituitary gland**, which is a bit like a thermostat regarding thyroid function. When the pituitary senses that the levels have dropped below normal, it will secrete TSH (thyroid stimulating hormone), which causes the thyroid to make more T3 and T4. Likewise when there are too many thyroid hormones, the pituitary acts by stopping production of TSH so that the levels return to normal. If your doctor suggests blood tests, he/she is looking to measure whether you are making too much or too little thyroid hormone.

Likewise, if you develop thyroid antibodies, this will indicate that you are developing an autoimmune disease of the thyroid, either Grave's Disease (hyperthyroidism) or Hashimoto's (hypothyroidism). Those who develop autoimmune thyroid disorders are more likely to develop other autoimmune diseases as well as other health problems.

A physical symptom to watch for that points specifically to an underactive thyroid, hypothyroidism, is that your eyebrows have thinned, and in particular, if the outer edge of the eyebrows have thinned or even disappeared that's a sign that it's time to have your thyroid checked.

The Parathyroid Glands

The parathyroid glands are actually unrelated to the thyroid itself *except* by location in the neck and the fact that they are part of the endocrine system. There are four parathyroid glands and they are responsible for controlling levels of calcium in the body. Calcium is the only mineral in the body with glands that control its levels.

When calcium levels get low the glands release a parathyroid hormone (PTH) to increase the concentration of calcium in the blood. When levels are too high, they stop producing the hormones so that calcium levels drop.

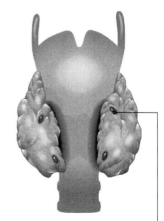

The Parathyroid Glands

Thymus Gland

The thymus gland lies beneath the top of the breastbone. It is divided into two lobes and is responsible for processing T-lymphocytes, which govern immunity in our cells, helping our cells to recognize invading bacteria, abnormal cell growth, and viruses. The thymus is also a critical organ of the lymphatic system. Without a thymus gland, we would have no resistance to disease.

When we have acute infection, the thymus gland can shrivel very quickly to half its size. It is most productive during puberty. Depending on diet and lifestyle, the thymus will shrink over the years of your life. In all of us, it will eventually shrink until it's barely detectable as we become elder. It is because of this that scientists once thought it had no purpose in adulthood. However, this has now been proven incorrect. It plays an important part in the development of immunity in our early lives.

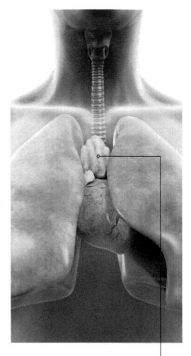

Thymus Gland

The adrenal glands are walnut-shaped and sit on the top of both kidneys. There are two parts, an inner **medulla** and an outer **cortex**, and each part secretes different hormones responsible for different actions. The adrenal glands interact with the hypothalamus and pituitary gland and the hypothalamus produces corticotropin-releasing hormones, which stimulate the pituitary gland.

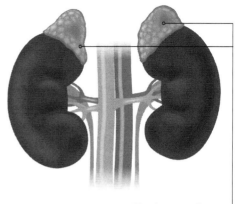

THE ADRENAL GLANDS

The pituitary gland, in response to the message, produces corticotropin hormones, which stimulate the adrenal glands to produce corticosteroid hormones. The hormones produced by the adrenal glands are part of the body's stress response and are essential for life.

The cortex secretes corticosteroids like hydrocortisone directly into the bloodstream. Hydrocortisone, also known as cortisol, controls the body's use of fats, proteins, and carbohydrates. The hormones secreted by the cortex have an effect on body functions such as metabolism, blood chemicals and characteristics of the body. Another hormone secreted by the cortex is corticosterone, which together with hydrocortisone hormones, suppresses inflammatory responses in the body and also affects the immune system. This process alone can help you understand why thyroid issues lead to weight and metabolism issues as well as poor pain management. One of the signs that my endocrine system was poorly functioning was a steady weight gain of twenty pounds despite the same real food diet and the same amount of exercise. Then my pain level went up and fatigue set in.

Other hormones secreted by the cortex include **aldosterone, androgen** and **testosterone**. Aldosterone controls the level of sodium excreted into the urine, thus maintaining blood volume and pressure; androgen is secreted in the female body, but circulates more during menopause. Testosterone is known as the "male" hormone, or androgen. It plays a key role in the development of male reproductive tissues, and characteristics such as increased muscle, bone mass, and the growth of body hair. In women it is often linked to sex drive.

The **medulla** secretes hormones to enable us to cope with stress. These hormones are **adrenaline** which increases heart rate and assists the flow of blood to the brain and muscles, reduces blood flow to the skin by producing sweat, assists in the conversion of glycogen to glucose in the liver which in turn raises blood sugar levels. This allows us to react appropriately when we are faced with danger or emergencies that call on us to perform at our best. **Noradrenaline** acts on receptors to stimulate the sympathetic nervous system, slows the heart rate and increases blood pressure.

What can go wrong? Like the other glands, problems can and do arise. Adrenal fatigue and autoimmune diseases like, Addison's disease and Cushing's syndrome, are on the rise. The symptoms of Addison's disease sound like other endocrine gland disorders such as weakness, fatigue, intolerance to the cold, muscular aches and pains, giddiness, and weight loss.

THE PANCREAS

The pancreas is part of the digestive system as well as the endocrine system. Remember I said all of our systems are connected! It is about six inches long and its position in the abdomen is roughly where your ribs join at the bottom of the sternum and it is behind the stomach and in close proximity to your liver.

It is divided into parts with the wide end called the "head", the thin end called the "tail" and the middle portion called the "body." It produces digestive enzymes which flow into the main pancreatic duct, as well as the hormones insulin, glucagon, and other digestive hormones like somatostatin and gastrin.

The part of the pancreas that produces digestive enzymes is called the exocrine pancreas and makes up most of the pancreas. The part dealing with hormones such as insulin and glucagon production is of course the endocrine pancreas.

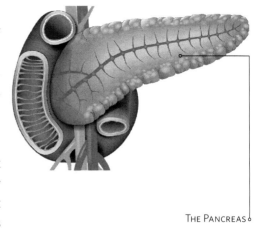

THE PANCREAS

The digestive system breaks down our food and after about two hours it moves into the duodenum, partially digested. Upon the arrival of food at the duodenum, the pancreas releases the enzymes to further digest the food until it is a lot smaller. Then it gets absorbed into the body by the small intestine.

The endocrine pancreas is responsible for insulin and glucagon production, which regulates blood sugar levels and keeps them stable. If the pancreas does not make enough insulin, then diabetes results. Blood sugar levels are regulated by the production of insulin, too high and the pancreas produces more insulin, too low and the pancreas releases less. Glucagon assists insulin in blood sugar regulation and is secreted when blood sugar is low and inhibited when blood sugar is high. It is basically the opposite of insulin. Excess glucagon production causes hyperglycemia.

Somatostatin is a hormone produced by many tissues in the body, principally in the nervous and digestive systems. It regulates a wide variety of physiological functions and inhibits the secretion of other hormones, the activity of the gastrointestinal tract and the rapid reproduction of normal and tumor cells. Somatostatin may also act as a neurotransmitter in the nervous system.

Somatostatin is also secreted by the pancreas in response to many factors related to food intake, such as high blood levels of glucose and amino acids. An overproduction of somatostatin may result in the suppression of insulin secretion from the pancreas leading to raised blood glucose levels (diabetes), the formation of gallstones, intolerance to fat in the diet, and diarrhea.

THE GONADS

The gonads—ovaries in females and testes in males—are responsible for producing the sex hormones of the body. These sex hormones determine the secondary sex characteristics of adult females and adult males. Testosterone is the primary androgen of the testes. The importance of testosterone is not limited to puberty.

Throughout adulthood, the hormone is integral in a variety of functions in males, such as maintaining libido, sperm production, maintaining muscle strength and mass, and promoting healthy bone density. For women, research reveals that sexual health is greatly affected by low testosterone levels. Low levels of this hormone in women can present as fatigue, vaginal dryness, weight gain, loss of muscle, mood swings, hair loss and more.

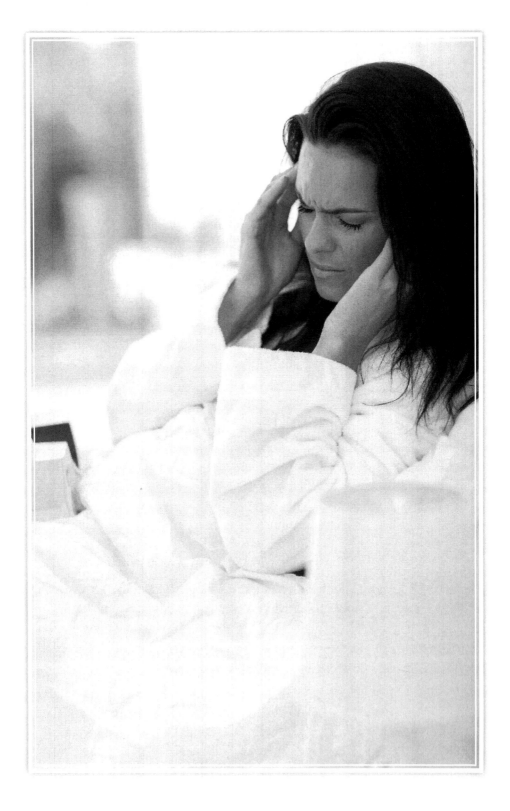

Common Disorder of the Endocrine System

Your thyroid releases hormones and is your chief gland of energy and metabolism. Every cell in your body has thyroid hormone receptors and your thyroid keeps your cells doing their job—breathing, body temperature control, heart rate, and weight management.

Hyperthyroidism is a condition in which the thyroid gland is overactive and makes excessive amounts of thyroid hormone. When the thyroid gland is overactive—*hyper*—the body's processes speed up and you may experience the following symptoms:

THE SYMPTOMS OF HYPERTHYROIDISM INCLUDE THE FOLLOWING:

- Fatigue or muscle weakness

- Hand tremors

- Mood swings

- Nervousness or anxiety

- Rapid heartbeat

- Heart palpitations or irregular heartbeat

- Skin dryness

- Trouble sleeping

- Weight loss

- Increased frequency of bowel movements

- Light periods or skipping periods

Causes of Hyperthyroidism

The thyroid gland makes the hormones thyroxine (T_4) and triiodothyronine (T_3) that play an important role in the way your whole body functions. If your thyroid gland makes too much T_4 and T_3, this is defined as hyperthyroidism.

The most common cause of hyperthyroidism is the autoimmune disorder Graves' disease. In this disorder, the body makes an antibody (a protein produced by the body to protect against a virus or bacteria) called thyroid-stimulating immunoglobulin (TSI) that causes the thyroid gland to make too much thyroid hormone. Graves' disease runs in families and is more commonly found in women.

Hyperthyroidism may also be caused by nodules in the thyroid gland that cause the thyroid to produce excessive amounts of thyroid hormones. In addition, inflammation of the thyroid gland—called thyroiditis—resulting from a virus or a problem with the immune system may temporarily cause symptoms of hyperthyroidism. Furthermore, some people who consume too much iodine may cause the thyroid gland to overproduce thyroid hormones. Pregnancy can trigger hyperthyroidism in some women as well.

Hypothyroidism, or underactive—*hypo*—thyroid function, is a silent epidemic. People can suffer for years with symptoms that our conventional medical system frequently misses because complaints seem scattered or vague and it can easily be mistaken as something else.

Hypothyroidism is a condition in which the body lacks sufficient thyroid hormone. Since the main purpose of thyroid hormone is to run the body's metabolism, it is understandable that people with this condition will have symptoms associated with a slow metabolism. The estimates vary, but approximately ten million Americans have this common medical condition. In fact, as many as ten percent of women may have some degree of thyroid hormone deficiency.

There are two fairly common causes of hypothyroidism. The first is a result of previous (or ongoing) inflammation of the thyroid gland, which leaves a large percentage of the cells of the thyroid damaged and incapable of producing sufficient hormone. The second, and most common, cause of thyroid gland failure is called autoimmune thyroiditis (Hashimoto's thyroiditis), a form of thyroid inflammation caused by your own immune system.

There are several other rare causes of hypothyroidism, one of them being a completely "normal," thyroid gland that is not making enough hormone because of a problem in the pituitary gland. If the pituitary does not produce enough thyroid stimulating hormone (TSH) then the thyroid simply does not have the signal to make hormone. So it doesn't.

- Fatigue

- Weakness

- Weight gain or increased difficulty losing weight

- Coarse, dry hair

- Dry, rough pale skin

- Hair loss

- Cold intolerance (you can't tolerate cold temperatures like those around you)

- Muscle cramps and frequent muscle aches

- Constipation

- Depression

- Irritability

- Memory loss

- Abnormal menstrual cycles

- Decreased libido

Each individual patient may have any number of these symptoms, and they will vary with the severity of the thyroid hormone deficiency and the length of time the body has been deprived of the proper amount of hormone.

In many cases, hypo- and hyper- thyroidism don't originate as a thyroid problem. They are immune system issues that are often overlooked by the medical community because as I mentioned, the symptoms can be vague and similar to other conditions. We also have the tendency to break the body apart into individual parts so the place many doctors start is the organ in question rather that the immune system which may be the trigger.

According to Dr. Datis Kharrazian, author of *Why Do I Still have Thyroid Symptoms? When My Lab Tests Are Normal*, ninety percent of people with hypothyroidism have Hashimoto's, an autoimmune hypothyroid condition, whereby the immune system attacks thyroid tissue. In hyperthyroidism, the autoimmune condition is Grave's disease. Therefore, to address thyroid disease, or any autoimmune condition, you have to get to the source of the imbalance. If we focus on treating symptoms alone we are allowing the condition to continue.

If you suspect you have hormonal issues creating other health problems, talk with your doctor. Be specific about your concerns and ask for tests that can rule out serious autoimmune disease or early warning signs. If your doctor refuses to hear your concerns or run tests to rule out hormone issues, find one who will.

- **24-HOUR CORTISOL SALIVA TEST:** An at-home test to evaluate your circadian cortisol levels at key times during a twenty-four-hour period.

- **DHEA:** Measured in conjunction with the twenty-four-hour adrenal cortisol saliva test. See above.

- **AB (ANTITHYROGLOBULIN):** Measures the level of the antibody protein antithyroglobulin in order to discern the presence of Hashimoto's disease.

- **B12:** Measures an essential vitamin, B12, which can be low in hypothyroid patients due to low stomach acid.

- **FREE T3:** Active thyroid hormone.

- **FREE T4:** Thyroid storage hormone.

- **REVERSE FREE T3:** The body produces the benign RT3 naturally to rid itself of excess of T4, but in some cases, such as high or low cortisol, it's made in excess and that excess clogs your cell receptors from receiving regular T3.

- **MAGNESIUM:** Thyroid patients can be chronically low in the magnesium, which causes a multitude of problems.

- **THYROID PEROXIDASE ANTIBODY (TPO):** Measures the thyroid antibody TPO, which will be above the normal level in the presence of Hashimoto's disease.

- **THRYOID STIMULATING HORMONE (TSH):** Measures the actual TSH in your body, a pituitary hormone messenger. The lab is using a pituitary hormone to tell you if you have a thyroid issue.

- **VITAMIN D:** 25-hydroxy vitamin D lab test measures the level of the hormone vitamin D, which plays a vital role in your immune system. 50–80 at the minimum is your range goal. Many thyroid patients are low in D due to digestive issues from being undiagnosed or undertreated, plus problems with celiac or non-celiac gluten intolerance, or absorption issues (dysbiosis).

- **FERRITIN:** Measures your levels of storage iron, which can be chronically low in hypothyroid patients.

In the meantime, keep exploring additional ways to care for yourself on a deeper level. Consider this book an opportunity to evaluate your current lifestyle and dietary habits and then experiment with ways you can improve your self-care.

Adrenal fatigue can affect you if you suffer from prolonged periods of stress or lack of sleep. Thyroid patients can also suffer from it, as can some other autoimmune disease sufferers. Although I was diagnosed with chronic fatigue syndrome, a closer look from a functional perspective and some specific lab tests showed it was in fact adrenal fatigue.

Adrenal fatigue can strike more than once. Below is a snapshot of my lab test years after my initial case of adrenal fatigue, which shows my cortisol levels well below the "low" range. So in the morning when my cortisol should be at its highest point in the day (that's what gets us up in the morning), I was not producing enough.

Functional Adrenal Stress Profile

PARAMETER	RESULT	REFERENCE RANGE	UNITS
Cortisol—Morning (6–8 AM)	9.4*	13.0–24.0	nM/L
Cortisol—Noon (12–1 PM)	3.3*	5.0–8.0	nM/L
Cortisol—Afternoon (4–5 PM)	2.8*	4.0–7.0	nM/L
Cortisol—Nighttime (10PM–12 AM)	1.0	1.0–3.0	nM/L
Cortisol Sum	16.5*	23.0–42.0	nM/L
DHEA-S Average	1.91*	2.00–10.00	ng/mL
Cortisol / DHEA-S Ratio	8.6*	5.0–6.0	Ratio

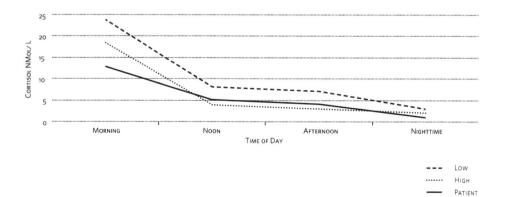

In addition, cortisol acts as an anti-inflammatory over autoimmune reactions, but when the levels of this hormone are insufficient to cope with the autoimmune reactions taking place, you can really suffer. My pain level was unbearable at times.

Adrenal fatigue is largely dismissed by the medical profession, who view it in a similar light to chronic fatigue syndrome. Many doctors assume it's all in the patient's head and I suppose after learning more about the endocrine system, there may be some truth to that, but not in the way they are thinking. Chronic fatigue syndrome and adrenal fatigue go hand in hand and can be reversed.

As Dr. James Wilson covers in his book *Adrenal Fatigue: The 21st Century Stress Syndrome*, stress can kill. The first of the three stages of adrenal fatigue he describes, is the *Alarm Reaction: A Fight or Flight Response*. This is your body's natural response to a threat. Our ancestors would have experienced this if a tiger chased them. Today, it might be a car accident or an unexpected death in the family.

Your body releases stress chemicals into the blood stream, like adrenaline. Your blood pressure rises, heart rate increases, and your breathing pattern changes, and your digestion slows down (blood is diverted away from skin and stomach). After this alarm phase your body goes into a short-term recovery stage that lasts approximately twenty-four to forty-eight hours. You can feel more tired after this over-expenditure of energy.

Sadly, today everyone seems to be in a chronic state of stress. When this happens, the body enters a phase of resistance, or stage two of adrenal fatigue. This is when you body continues to fight long after the "fight-or-flight" response is needed. When this continues over a long period of time, people move into stage three, exhaustion. I also call this failure to adapt. Everything is affected. Pregnenalone, the precursor to all hormones, is needed by the body to produce sex hormones, like estrogen, testosterone and progesterone. When the body is suffering with adrenal fatigue it begins to "steal" pregnenolone, in an effort to make more cortisol. This depletes your pregnenolone, which impacts your body's ability to produce estrogen, testosterone, and progesterone. Ultimately, you end up with little to no interest in sex. This is not your fault. It is a real issue for so many people and rather than shake it off as getting older or being too tired from the kids, I would encourage you to consider what's really going on inside and get the support you need to turn it around.

The final stage of adrenal fatigue is Addison's disease. This is an autoimmune condition when the immune system attacks the adrenal glands and the glands no longer produce the hormones needed for the body's response to stress. It is a medical emergency.

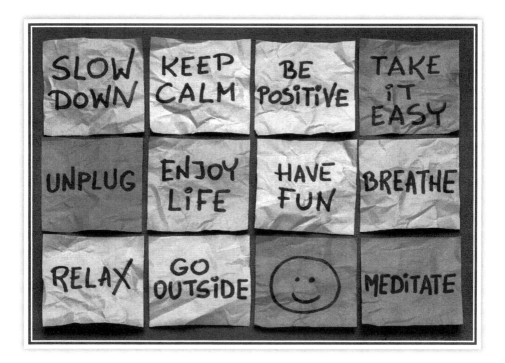

As with all autoimmune diseases, the cause for the autoimmune attack is unknown and in some cases can be caused by viral infections, fungal infections and tumors. Some long-term medications can also be responsible for both long-term and temporary loss of function referred to as secondary adrenal suppression, such as those to treat bowel disease and asthma. Steroidal drugs can also do this.

The adrenals assist in our body's ability to cope with stress, whether this stress is financial, relationships, drug abuse and addictions, labor, illness, work, bereavement, or even environmental triggers. No matter how mild or severe the stress, being individual to each person and their ability to cope, the adrenals and their hormones play a critical role.

Also if you suffer from a chronic illness, the adrenals are put under additional stress, sometimes critical. This causes their hormone output to be diminished. Although they still work, they don't work well enough to maintain health. The occurrence of adrenal fatigue can vary from a temporary bout to a lifetime if the symptoms are not identified and treated.

The symptoms of adrenal fatigue sound familiar to thyroid disease in some ways with the persistent tiredness, feeling emotionally overwhelmed, and being unable to cope with situations. This can build up until we can't cope with anything at all.

It also includes that inability to get up in the mornings no matter how much you've slept (try sleeping in with three little boys), low immune response and inability to recover from viruses and minor illnesses to persistent mouth ulcers and infections. This is exactly what was happening to me. It was always blamed on my fibromyalgia and I was told to cope with it.

Also keep in mind that seemingly unrelated issues like tooth problems are a result of adrenal fatigue. From tooth abscesses to gum infection to mercury filling these things can all suppress cortisol production. Sometimes adrenal fatigue can be as a direct result of poor dental work or mercury amalgams. Do not use mercury amalgams fillings in your mouth. Your dentist can use composite filling that is safe and effective. If your dentist insists on mercury, find a new dentist.

If you have mercury fillings and you suspect they are contributing to your autoimmune disease, chronic illness, or adrenal fatigue, find a holistic dentist specifically trained in the safe removal of mercury.

OTHER SYMPTOMS TO LOOK FOR INCLUDE:

- HIGH OR LOW BLOOD PRESSURE: Low blood pressure can often have the symptom of light-headedness.

- FOOD CRAVINGS AND WEIGHT CHANGES: Weight gain in the abdomen and thighs and cravings for salty or sugary foods (sometimes feeling uncontrollable).

- ENERGY OR LACK THERE OF: Unable to stop, always on speed forward; or ongoing fatigue, lack of stamina, feeling tired and wired much of the time. Always feeling unmotivated.

- INABILITY TO COPE OR FOCUS: Feeling overwhelmed most of the time, very short fuse, anxiety attacks; fuzzy thinking, inability to stay focused on one task.

- IMMUNE: Frequent infections, longer recovery from illness or infections.

- SLEEP: Inability to fall asleep or waking throughout the night, sound sleep but waking exhausted.

Many other conditions can overlap the above symptoms and adrenal fatigue may not be the root cause. It can, however, be a co-existing condition and supporting the adrenal glands is important for overall health.

Dietary triggers: The foods that may be hurting you

Most people think of food as pleasure or a form of celebration, which it is. As the saying goes, "A party without a cake is just a meeting." But what if food becomes harmful? The number of food allergies is rapidly increasing with effects from mild rashes to migraines and even in some cases full metabolic dysfunction.

Food sensitivities and intolerances, on the other hand, are commonly misunderstood and often go unrecognized. The writings of Hippocrates dating back to 400 B.C. discuss the role of adverse foods reactions in the development of many health complaints. However, it wasn't until the twentieth century that formal research began documenting food allergies in scientific journals.

The reason food allergies, sensitivities, and intolerances are so important is because foods are linked to many disorders. The problem is that ninety percent of the people with food reactions never experience digestive complaints and therefore don't relate the foods we eat to common health issues. Eating food is something we all do multiple times a day. Shockingly, it is almost always the last place people look when exploring the potential cause of their health issues. I was no different.

To better understand food sensitivities and the potential dangers of missing them, it is helpful to understand the difference and similarities between allergies, sensitivities and intolerances.

Allergies

An allergic reaction is an immune response to a foreign substance (an antigen) that results in inflammation and organ dysfunction. Allergens can be chemical, food, or environmental. In people with allergies or sensitivities, an immediate or delayed adverse reaction by the immune system can occur even when other people have no reaction to the same food or environmental trigger.

What's really going on in there?

A food allergy is an antigen-antibody response to a particular food (IgG or IgE are the usual antibodies involved) and most often the reaction is immediate—within two hours after exposure. IgE-mediated reaction is mainly seen in airborne allergies like pollens, weeds, and dust. These antibodies attach to mast cells and are mainly found in the air passages, blood and skin. When an allergen enters the body, the mast cells release histamine to ward off the allergen. Often anaphylactic shock, wheezing, hives, rash, swelling, panic attacks, or difficulty swallowing can take place. Personally, I know this all too well as my youngest son, Treyson, has a severe allergy to peanuts and the proteins found in the saliva and skin of dogs and cats.

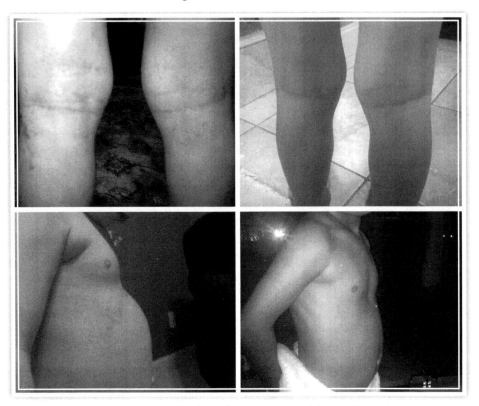

(Left) Treyson's eczema and abdominal swelling from pasteurized-commercial dairy and GMO grains. (Right) Removal of offending foods and gut healing.

SENSITIVITY

A sensitivity reaction is also an immune response to a chemical, food, or environmental element. In people with sensitivities, a delayed-adverse reaction by the immune system is more common and can occur even when other people have no reaction to the same food or environmental trigger.

WHAT'S REALLY GOING ON IN THERE?

A delayed reaction, also known as "masked" food allergy, can occur up to seventy-two hours after exposure to the antigen. What? Yes, you read that correctly. It can take up to three days after the food is eaten to feel an immune reaction. This delayed reaction makes it extremely difficult to pin point the food. It is one of the primary reasons I believe people rarely consider food as the trigger.

- Dark circles under the eyes or puffy eyes
- Fluid retention
- Dermatitis
- Asthma
- Joint pain or inflammation
- Mood swings or irritability
- Indigestion, pain or discomfort
- Headaches

- Chronic ear infections
- Poor memory or "foggy" brain
- Anxiety and/or depression
- Neurological symptoms
- Fatigue
- Restlessness or waking at night
- Gas, bloating or stomach distention

For a complete list of possible symptoms associated with food sensitivities please see page 62.

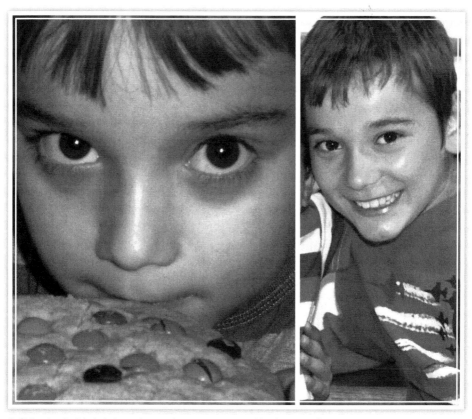

(Left) Stephen had dark circles under eyes (common symptom of food sensitivity).
(Right) Removal off offending foods and gut healing.

POSSIBLE SYMPTOMS ASSOCIATED WITH FOOD SENSITIVITIES

- Abdominal pain
- Abdominal swelling
- ADD
- ADHD
- Aggressive Behavior
- Airborne Allergies
- Anxiety
- Arthritis
- Asthma
- Athlete's Foot/Fungus
- Autism
- Bacterial Infection
- Bloating
- Bronchitis
- Burping
- Candida/yeast
- Colitis/Ulcerative Colitis
- Confusion
- Constipation
- Crohn's

- Depression
- Dermatitis
- Diabetes 1
- Diabetes 2
- Diarrhea
- Eczema
- Failure to gain weight
- Fatigue
- Fevers
- Fibromyalgia
- Frequent Infections
- Fuzzy thinking
- Gas
- General Food Intolerances
- Hashimoto's
- Hay Fever
- Headaches
- Heartburn/reflux
- Hyperthyroid
- Hypothyroid

- Infertility
- Insomnia
- Irritable bowel (IBS)
- Join Pain
- Mood Swings
- Mouth Sores
- Multiple Sclerosis
- Muscle pain
- Nervousness
- Obesity
- Osteoporosis
- Parasites
- Poor memory
- Recurrent Colds and Flu
- Shortness of Breath
- Sinus/Nasal Congestion
- Urinary Tract Infections
- Weight Gain
- Weight loss resistance

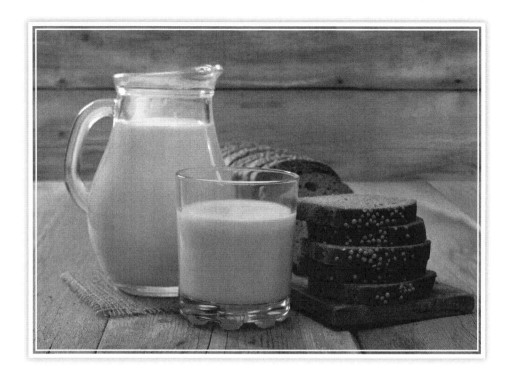

ALTHOUGH ANY FOOD CAN TRIGGER A NEGATIVE RESPONSE IN THE BODY, THE MOST COMMON FOODS INCLUDE:

- Gluten

- Dairy

- Soy

- Corn

- Sugar

Food sensitivities are estimated to affect millions of people. Some practitioners suggest as many as sixty percent of Americans have unrecognized food reactions. We can expect that number to increase given the rapid trend of genetically modified foods, over consumption of processed foods and our dependency on medications.

While lab tests can be useful (I'll cover that later), the best, most accurate and economical way to determine if you have any food sensitivities is with an Elimination diet. This will tell you something the lab test will not, which is how YOUR body reacts to foods more specifically.

When it comes to allergies and food sensitivities and their role in chronic disease or autoimmunity, we must look at the immune system rather than symptoms of the organs or system of the body that troubles us. Recognize that foods can be an immune "trigger" leading to chronic inflammation and ultimately chronic disease. If we remove the trigger and support, not suppress, the immune system, we can support our body's natural ability to heal. While there is no known cure for autoimmune conditions, the functional approach takes into account the whole body and works to bring balance to all systems of the body with the understanding that the body works in symmetry.

INTOLERANCES AND OTHER FOOD REACTIONS

Another type of adverse food reaction is called food intolerance. Food intolerance is an umbrella term that refers to any abnormal response to a food that is not caused by an antibody/antigen reaction. For example, some food intolerances are caused by enzyme deficiencies, while others are caused by poor function of the digestive tract or a reaction to a natural or synthetic chemical.

LACTOSE INTOLERANCE

You may be most familiar with lactose intolerance, which affects as many as thirty percent of American adults, and is particularly common in people of African and Asian heritage.

People with lactose intolerance do not produce enough of the digestive enzyme called lactase, which breaks down the milk sugar (lactose) found in dairy products. When too much undigested lactose makes its way into the large intestine, people suffer from gas and/or diarrhea.

Keep in mind that lactose intolerance is not the same as dairy allergy or sensitivity to the protein in dairy called casein. Dairy is a controversial health food in nutrition. According to our government, dairy should be a staple in the diet however, the Journal of American Medicine admits there is little to no evidence to support the health claims like bone health. To the contrary, dairy sensitivities are often linked to eczema, hormone disorders, acne and even increased risks of osteoporosis. There are people that tolerate, even thrive, on dairy. The key is to find out if you're one of the few. If so, quality matters most. Many people experience digestive and other health problems when they consume pasteurized milk, but have no issues with raw milk. The Weston A. Price Foundation conducted an informal survey of over 700 families, and determined that over eighty percent of those diagnosed with lactose intolerance no longer suffer from symptoms after switching to raw milk.

Food Additives

Synthetic food colorings, including food dyes, Blue #1, Blue #2, Red #3 and Red #40, Yellow #6 and Yellow # 5 (tartrazine), are problematic for many people, especially chil-

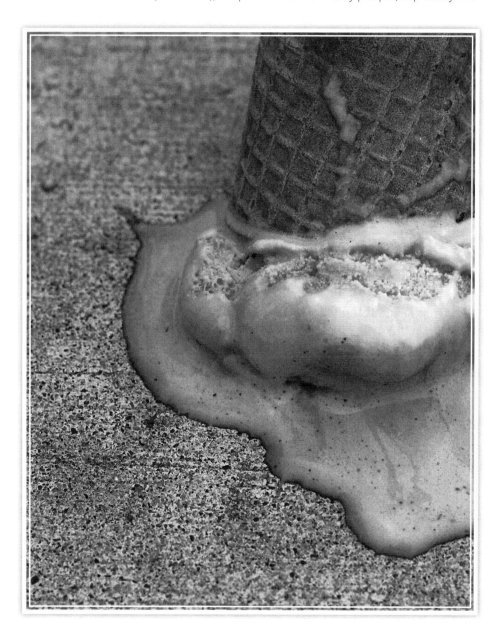

dren. They may contribute to behavioral problems, ADD and ADHD. Synthetic food colorings come in almost everything that appeals to kids today like colored ice pops, ice cream, macaroni and cheese, candy, fruit drinks, yogurts and more.

Monosodium glutamate (MSG) is used as a flavor enhancer particularly in many foods. Glutamate itself is a naturally occurring amino acid found in many protein-rich foods, including cheese, milk, meat, walnuts, mushrooms and broccoli. This amino acid is also produced by the body and used in metabolism. However, this is not the same as *free* glutamate found in processed foods. Free glutamate is made by fermenting starch, corn, sugar beets, molasses, or sugar cane to "free" naturally occurring glutamate. Free Glutamate affects the neurological pathways of the brain. In the late 1960s, people began connecting their "Asian restaurant headache" with having eaten food with MSG. Children with autism, ADD and ADHD symptoms are often reacting to MSG in their diet. Many people report disorientation, depression and fatigue from consuming MSG. MSG is blamed for a range of serious neurological and physiological disorders. Studies have identified both MSG and aspartame as excitotoxins, substances that over-stimulate the neurotransmitters to the point of cell damage.

MSG is also blamed, in part, for the obesity epidemic. John W. Olney, M.D. published a study in which he found that monosodium glutamate, given to mice, resulted in obesity and other neuroendocrine disorders due to lesions in the arcuate nucleus of the hypothalamus.[25] In studies around the world, scientists create obese mice and rats to use in diet or diabetes test studies by injecting them with MSG.

Hidden Sources of MSG:

- Natural flavorings
- Bouillon cubes
- Hydrolyzed Vegetable Protein
- Hydrolyzed Plant Protein
- Autolyzed Plant Protein
- Sodium Caseinate

- Calcium Caseinate
- Textured Protein
- Yeast Extract
- Autolyzed Yeast
- Vegetable Protein Extract
- Gelatin

Aspartame is known to affect intelligence. It is a toxic chemical and should not be consumed as part of a healthy diet. Aspartame is commonly found in sugar-free foods, gums, soda, toothpaste, cereal, drink mixes, and more. Dr. Russell Blaylock, neurosurgeon and author of *Excitotoxins: The Taste That Kills You*, said, "Aspartame stimulates the neurons of the brain to death, causing brain damage of varying degrees."[26] Dr. H.J. Roberts, diabetic specialist and world expert on aspartame poisoning, tells how aspartame poisoning is escalating Alzheimer's disease.

High Fructose Corn Syrup (HFCS) is one of the worst additives/ingredients on the market today. This highly-refined artificial sweetener is not so sweet after all. It is made from genetically-modified corn crops. Nothing packs on the pounds quite like HFCS.[27] There is also a strong link between the consumption of high fructose corn syrup and elevated triglyceride and LDL (bad cholesterol) levels.[28]

Sodium Sulphite (sulfites): Many people are also unable to tolerate sulfites that appear in abundance in our food supply. These sulfur-containing preservatives are used in dried fruits, wines, and many other processed foods. According to the FDA, it is estimated that one in one hundred people can't tolerate sulfites. The most common symptoms related to sulfite sensitivity are asthma, breathing difficulty, headaches and rashes.

Sulfur dioxide is a type of sulfite, a preservative whose name might be more familiar. Even a small amount of sulfite can wreak health havoc if you're sensitive to it. If you have asthma, sulfite sensitivity is very common and eating dried fruits could cause serious health issues, including breathing problems. If you have asthma, you have a much higher risk of developing a reaction to sulfur dioxide than a person without asthma. By contrast, if you don't have asthma, you have a very low risk of having sulfite sensitivity.

Carrageenan is considered a natural additive extracted from specific red seaweed. These seaweeds are then processed with alkali to be used as a natural food additive. However, when the seaweed is processed with acid instead of alkali, the carrageenan is "degraded" (lower weight) and can also be called poligeenan. Some scientists believe degraded carrageenan in our food is not safe due to possible intestinal damage like lesions, ulceration, and gastrointestinal inflammation. Degraded carrageenan is commonly used to induce inflammation in laboratory animals. The good news is, it's not allowed in our food. The bad new is, some scientists believe the food grade carrageenan, that is the natural additive processed with alkali, is also a concern. Some believe the acid in our stomach may "degrade" it.

Carrageenan is used as a substitute for fat in low fat products or as non-dairy replacements. It has no nutritional value or flavor. Its main use is a stabilizer for beverages that separate so the consumer does not have to shake it. It can also be used in deli meat or prepared foods, like chicken, when the brine includes carrageenan to improve tenderness. Fortunately, many health conscious companies are removing it from their products.

Phenols are naturally occurring chemicals present in food dyes, artificial flavors, preservatives, fruits, and vegetables. Almost all foods have phenols, but in varying amounts. Salicylates are a subgroup of phenols.

Salicylates are naturally-occurring in many vegetables, herbs, spices, fruits, and chocolate. Salicylates are produced by plants to serve as their own natural protection from diseases, insects, fungi, and harmful bacteria. However, these naturally-occurring components in plant foods have been associated with a variety of health issues.

Salicylates are chemically very similar to the man-made chemical acetylsalicylic acid, more commonly known as aspirin. So if you are sensitive to aspirin, you may want to explore your reaction to salicylates in foods.

When the body has the correct levels of sulphates and liver enzymes, phenols are easily metabolized. The body utilizes what it needs from the chemicals and properly disposes of the rest through the bowels. In those whose levels may not be adequate, for example those with leaky gut syndrome or low levels of sulfur in the body (common among people with autoimmune, especially autism), an intolerance to this chemical family can occur rather quickly. Think of it as the cup spilling over. When the body accumulates too many phenols and lacks the ability to clear them from the body, the reaction occurs. But remember, this is not an allergy, it's an intolerance.

Some people with gut issues such as yeast/bacteria overgrowth can develop salicylate intolerance as a result of the existing gut damage. When this happens the body tries to get rid of them by triggering an immune system response. Because phenols are so common in healthy foods, a person with a leaky gut will have much higher than normal levels of these chemicals in their blood and can very quickly develop an intolerance.

Salicylates stimulate the central nervous system in people who react to them. This can often bring with it an emotionally extreme high followed by an extreme low— just like people who eat too much sugar and then crash. Some people feel extremely agitated and even angry. There is no question that my three-year old son has a low threshold for phenols. If he eats a handful of grapes or blueberries, look out!

Reactions to the phenol family can include: dark circles under the eyes, red face or ears, diarrhea, headache, difficulty falling asleep at night, night waking, and in some cases excessively tired and lethargic. Behavioral symptoms of a reaction can be: hyperactivity, aggression, head banging or other self-injury, and even inappropriate laughter. Hyperactivity is more common in children's reactions where as adults generally experience symptoms similar to chronic fatigue.

The tough part is that phenols, and more specifically salicylates, are found in most foods that we eat—especially the healthy ones. So it is almost impossible to completely eliminate them from your diet. The most realistic thing to do is try to only eat the foods that contain smaller amounts of the chemical and rotate the foods in your diet to avoid a build-up. In addition to those mentioned above, salicylate sensitivity can present as follows:

- Stomach pain/upset or nausea

- Tinnitus (ringing of the ears)

- Itchy skin, hives or rashes (Urticaria)

- Asthma or other breathing difficulties

- Headaches

- Swelling of hands, feet, face, lips or eyelids

- Bed wetting or urgency to pass water

- Persistent or nagging cough

- Changes in skin color/skin discoloration

- Sore, itchy, puffy or burning eyes

- Fatigue

- Sinusitis or nasal polyps

- Diarrhea

- Hyperactivity (especially in children)

- Poor concentration or memory loss

- Mood swings or agitation

Here is a list of foods that fall into the High to Very High category combined. To see a list of foods in the low to moderate categories, visit www.salicylatesensititivy.com

Foods High in Salicylates

HIGH	VERY HIGH	
FRUITS		
Apples	All dried fruit	Grapes
Grapefruit	Apricot	Guava
Kiwi	Avocado	Orange
Mandarin	Blackberry	Pineapple
Melons	Blackcurrant	Plum
Mulberry	Blueberry	Prune
Nectarine	Cantaloupe	Raisin
Peach	Cherries	Raspberry
Watermelon	Cranberry	Red currant
	Currant	Strawberry
	Dates	Tangerine
VEGETABLES		
Alfalfa sprouts	Canned green olives	
Artichoke	Chicory	
Broccoli	Chili peppers	
Canned black olives	Endive	
Cucumber	Hot pepper	
Eggplant	Peppers	
Fresh spinach	Pickles	
Okra	Radish	
Sweet potato	Water chestnut	
Watercress	Zucchini	
MEAT		
Pre-made gravies	Processed Lunch meats	
Some canned fish	Seasoned meats (salami, sausages, hotdogs)	
NUTS AND SEEDS		
Brazil nuts	Almond	
Macadamia nuts	Peanuts (with skin on)	
Pine nuts		
Pistachio		

SWEETS		
Chewing gum	Liquorice	
Honey	Mint flavored sweets	
Honey flavors	Peppermints	
Jam (except pear)		

FATS AND OILS	
Sesame oil	Coconut oil
Walnut oil	Olive oil

CONDIMENTS/SPICES		
All spice	Aniseed	Mint
Bay leaf	Basil	Nutmeg
Caraway	Black pepper	Oregano
Cardamom	Cayenne	Paprika
Cloves	Celery powder	Peppermint
Coriander	Chili flakes	Rosemary
Ginger	Chili powder	Sage
Mixed herbs	Cider vinegar	Tabasco
Pimiento	Cumin	Tarragon
	Curry	Thyme
	Dill	Turmeric
	Fenugreek	White pepper
	Tomato paste	White vinegar
	Ginger	Wine vinegar
	Honey	Worcester sauce
	Jams/jelly (commercial)	

BEVERAGES	
Regular coffee	
All teas	
Cordials and fruit flavored drinks	
Fruit and vegetable juices	
Liquor	
Port	
Wine	
Rum	

Most people are not familiar with nightshades. They are not the latest trend in eyewear. Nightshades are a botanical family of plants, technically called Solanaceae. If you suffer with arthritis or an arthritis-related disease such as lupus, rheumatism, and other musculoskeletal pain disorders, nightshades could be the problem.

These plants all contain cholinesterase inhibiting glycoalkaloids and steroid alkaloids. In animal studies, the glycoalkaloids in potatoes are known to contribute to irritable bowel syndrome (IBS) and negatively affect intestinal permeability but also muscle aches, pains and inflammation. According to Dr. Marvin Childers, "When these inhibitors accumulate in the body, alone or with other cholinesterase inhibitors such as caffeine or food impurities containing systemic cholinesterase inhibiting pesticides, the result may be a paralytic-like muscle spasm, aches, pains, tenderness, inflammation, and stiff body movements."[29, 30]

Here is a partial list of the most common nightshades:

- Bell peppers (sweet peppers)
- Cocoa
- Eggplant
- Hot peppers (such as chili peppers, jalapenos, habaneros, chili-based spices, red pepper, cayenne)
- Paprika
- Pepinos
- Pimentos
- Potatoes (but not sweet potatoes)
- Tomatoes
- Cayenne pepper
- Ashwagandha
- Goji berries
- Tobacco

Although not truly nightshades, blueberries, goji berries and ashwaganda (an adaptogenic herb) all share the same inflammation-inducing alkaloids. Other things to consider:

- Vodka (made from potatoes)
- Prescription or over the counter medication (can include starches or herbs)
- Baking products, especially gluten free processed food (often includes potato starch)

Arthritis is the most common disability in the United States affecting almost fifty million Americans. Osteoarthritis appears to be connected to the long-term consumption of the nightshade vegetables. According to a 2011 report by the Institute of Medicine of the National Academies appropriately titled *"Relieving Pain in America"*, an estimated 116 million adults live with chronic pain, which costs the United States $635 billion annually in health care and lost productivity.[31] So this begs the question: How many of these people are suffering from nightshade related pain?

If you are one of those people that feel you have "tried everything" for your arthritis with no results, it may be worth considering if nightshades are adversely affecting your health. Avoid nightshades for a three-month period and then reintroduce these foods and make note of any symptoms of pain, inflammation, stiffness or loss of energy. Symptoms may dissipate in a few hours or days if ingestion of the offending food is stopped, but this is based on the your sensitivity, the amount of nightshades consumed, and your level of inflammation.

Soy

Soy is a controversial "health" food in the nutrition industry. Popular among vegans and vegetarians, soy is often a main source of protein. However, you may be surprised to learn that soy is not a complete protein. Like all legumes, soybeans are deficient in sulfur-containing amino acids methionine and cystine. Plus, modern processing denatures fragile lysine.

Soy is also considered one of the top seven allergens and moving up the list to the top four quickly. It is also one of the highest genetically modified crops in the United States. Soy contains a high level of phytic acid and phytoestrogens (think hormones), which withdraws nutrients from the body when digested. For example, many soy eaters have low zinc levels due to the phytic acid. Diets high in phytic acid can cause growth problems in children too.

Soy isoflavones have been linked to endocrine disruption, infertility, breast cancer, hypothyroidism, and thyroid cancer. Soy was removed from our home after my husband developed gynecomastia, a common endocrine disorder in which there is a benign enlargement of breast tissue in males, on one side of his chest. My husband stands 6'2" tall with a lean athletic build so enlarged breast tissue was both noticeable and alarming. After ruling out breast cancer with a mammogram, surgery was the recommend treatment to remove the benign tumor. I suspected soy. My husband questioned the doctor about the potential role of food, which was met with an adamant "No". Not surprisingly, there were reported cases of soy and gynecomastia,[32] but they are outnumbered by ones disputing the relationship. We experimented anyway. I can tell you without a doubt that the removal of soy from my husband's diet resulted in a one hundred percent reversal of gynecomastia in less than three months. He has no enlarged tissue and no tumor. That's enough evidence for me.

It doesn't take much to impact your health. At the time of my husband's diagnosis we were eating tofu about once per week and an occasional servings of edamame (soybeans) in stir fry plus small amounts of soy in processed foods. Even just eating as little as 40 mg of soy isoflavones (approx. 30g of soy protein) can result in weight gain, fatigue and hypothyroidism.

The thyroid is also vulnerable to soy in the diet. This gland needs zinc to function normally and soy isoflavones deactivates thyroid peroxides, which is the enzyme needed to break down iodine and support thyroid hormone production. Other vitamins that get depleted with soy consumption are B12 and vitamin C.

There is also a misconception about the consumption of soy in Asia. Many people think soy is a staple in the Asian diet, however the average consumption of soy foods in China is ten grams (about two teaspoons) per day and up to sixty grams in parts of Japan. Asians consume soy foods in small amounts as a condiment, and not as a replacement for animal foods. They also consume fermented soy to neutralize toxins in soybeans unlike many of the modern soy foods found in our grocery stores shelves. These foods are not fermented and are processed in a way that denatures proteins.

Avoiding soy in the food supply is getting challenging for the average consumer. The following items are only a partial list of the many foods that has hidden sources of soy:

- Bread crumbs, cereals and crackers

- Hydrolyzed plant protein and hydrolyzed vegetable protein

- Imitation dairy food

- Infant formula, nutrition supplements for toddlers and children

- Meal replacements

- Bacon bits

There is even a lawsuit in Illinois, where convicts have gone to court claiming that too much soy in their diets has resulted in severe health problems, including heart

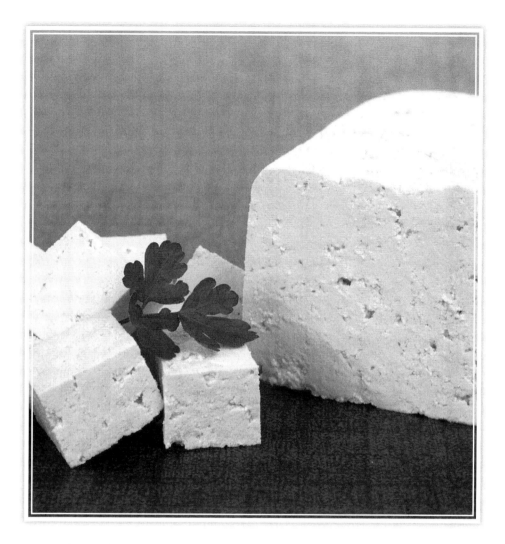

issues, thyroid damage, allergic reactions and gastrointestinal distress.[33] Due to the controlled environment in this case, it is easy to determine the amount of soy they were eating (estimated at one hundred grams per day) and the health outcomes. The prisoners served as a huge human experiment.

Not all soy is created equal. Fermentation deactivates the anti-nutrients that make soy more digestible. Also, most people are unlikely to eat high quantities of fermented soy as compared to drinking a large soy mochaccino or swapping real turkey for a dish of "tofurkey." If you do enjoy soy, best to stick to organic fermented versions like natto, tempeh, or miso.

To learn more about soy, I recommend *The Whole Soy Story,* by Dr. Kaayla Daniel, Ph.D.

The Silent Killers: Gluten and GMOs

Gluten

Technically, there is no such thing as "gluten"—if that word is being used to describe any single substance or even category of substances. The term gluten comes from the world of food industry, not science, and is applied to the combination of the prolamin proteins called gliadin and glutelins found in wheat.

Gluten is a gummy, yellow-gray material found in baked goods, that is left over after dough made from flour and water has been washed. When the dough is washed, many of the water-soluble substances and starches are washed off and what's left is a mixture that has traditionally been referred to as gluten.

If you were to dry out a ball of gluten it would measure to be about eighty percent protein by weight. The other twenty percent of this weight is made up of fats, carbohydrates, and minerals.

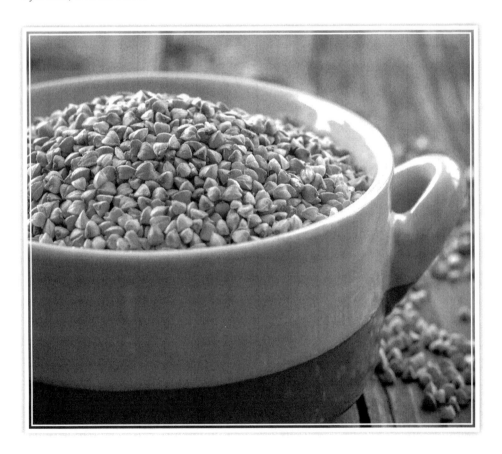

The Four Primary Gluten Proteins

There are four primary types of gluten proteins: 1) albumins, 2) globulins, 3) prolamins, and 4) glutelins. Glutelins have a more specific name when they are found in wheat. In this case, they are called glutenins. The prolamin proteins found in wheat are the gliadin proteins; in oats, they are avenins; in corn they are zeins; in rye they are secalins; and in barley they are hordeins.

Gluten is found in the following grains:

- Wheat
- Barley
- Bulgur
- Spelt

- Rye
- Kamut
- Triticale
- Semolina

- Pumpernickel
- Faro
- Oats (due to cross-contamination)

Gluten is sometimes referred to as *seitan* (wheat meat) in recipes.

Gluten is not in the following:

- Rice (all varieties)
- Buckwheat (part of the rhubarb family)
- Teff
- Amaranth

- Quinoa
- Corn
- Millet

Food additives are often potential hidden sources of gluten. These include:

- Dextrin, an incompletely hydrolyzed starch that may be derived from the dry heating of corn, potato, rice, tapioca, arrowroot, or wheat

- Caramel color, which can be made from heat treatment of many food-grade carbohydrates, including molasses, corn sugar, invert sugar, milk sugar, barley, malt syrup, or wheat starch hydrolysates

- Extracts, including vanillin extract, which often use grain alcohol in preparation of the extract and contain wheat protein residues

For a complete list of hidden sources of gluten see page 106.

Celiac disease is when there is an immune response to a specific epitope of gliadin (alpha-gliadin) and a specific type of transglutaminase (tTG-2). However, within the gliadin class, there are four different epitopes—alpha, beta, gamma, and omega—as well as other types of transglutaminase, like type 3 (found in the skin) and type 6 (found in the brain). Hang in there you'll see why this is important.

When we test for celiac disease or gluten intolerance most conventional labs only screen for antibodies to alpha-gliadin and transglutaminase-2. If you are reacting to any other part of the protein (and many people do), you will test negative for celiac disease and gluten intolerance despite the severity of your reaction to gluten or wheat.

Current statistics tell us that celiac disease affects about 1 in 100 people, or three million Americans. But considering the poor quality of conventional testing and the amount of people going undiagnosed, I suspect this number is much higher. Celiac disease is an autoimmune response to wheat proteins and transglutaminase enzymes in the gut. The consumption of wheat results in damage to the villi (the shag-like threads lining the small intestines). Once the villi are damaged, the body can no longer absorb nutrients.

Non-celiac gluten sensitivity (NCGS) is the new kid on the block. The reactions to gluten intolerance can affect nearly every tissue in the body, including the brain, skin, stomach, muscles, joints, hormones, and more. And it's not just a few who suffer; it's millions. Far more people have gluten sensitivity than you think—especially those who are chronically ill. Gluten sensitivity is even more common and some estimate may be as high as one in twenty Americans. And while most medical doctors continue to deny it exists, there are numerous studies to validate its existence including double-blind, placebo-controlled trials. And, if you're still not convinced join the millions of people around the world who are living with it, including me.

So why don't we hear much about it? Actually we do. Celiac disease and non-celiac gluten sensitivity are disguised as dozens of "other" diseases. In a recent article by Mark Hyman, M.D., titled *"Gluten: What You Don't Know Might Kill You,"*[34] he cites a review paper published in *The New England Journal of Medicine,* which lists fifty-five "diseases" that can be caused by eating gluten.[35] These include osteoporosis, irritable bowel disease, inflammatory bowel disease, anemia, cancer, fatigue, canker sores, and rheumatoid arthritis, lupus, multiple sclerosis, cerebellum ataxia and almost all other autoimmune diseases. Gluten is also linked to many psychiatric[36] and neurological diseases, including anxiety, depression,[37] schizophrenia,[38] dementia,[39] migraines, epilepsy, and neuropathy (nerve damage).[40] It has also been linked to autism.[41]

We used to think that gluten sensitivity or celiac disease was limited to people who had diarrhea or children with "failure to thrive". Now we know so much more. Gluten sensitivity causes an immune response in the body that creates inflammation throughout the body, with wide-ranging effects across all organ systems. It can be the single cause behind many different diseases. As Dr. Hyman says, "To correct these diseases, you need to treat the cause—which is often gluten sensitivity—not just the symptoms."

Of course, that doesn't mean that all autoimmune or chronic disease cases are caused by gluten in everyone—but it is important to look for it if you have any chronic illness. I agree with Dr. Hyman, "Health problems caused by gluten sensitivity cannot be treated with better medication. They can only be resolved by eliminating one hundred percent of the gluten from your diet."

The best way to test your reaction to gluten is with the elimination diet (see Section III of this book for details). If symptoms improve during the elimination period and return when gluten is reintroduced, you can assume NCGS is present. Or, a healthcare practitioner can order a comprehensive blood test (Array #3) from Cyrex Labratories, which screens for wheat and gluten proteins and transglutaminase enzymes, which can be helpful. I still recommend the elimination diet as the most accurate form of testing.

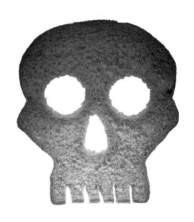

So why are we so sensitive to these "amber waves of grain?" The possible reasons include: One, we lack of genetic adaptation to grains in our diet. Wheat was introduced into Europe during the Middle Ages, and thirty percent of people of European descent carry the gene for celiac disease (HLA DQ2 or HLA DQ8),[42] which increases susceptibility to health problems from eating gluten; Two, American strains of wheat have significantly higher gluten content than those traditionally found in Europe;[43] And three, the use of glyphosate, an herbicide used by farmers to control weeds and dry down wheat, rice, sugarcane, and other crops just before harvest, results in gut damage and an increased risk of disease and food sensitivities.[44]

The Disturbing Truth

"Genetically modified organisms," or GMOs, are plants and animals that have been created by combining DNA of different species in a way that does not occur in nature to make them weather and pest resistant. Basically, you take the gene from one species (bacteria, virus, human) and force it into the DNA of other species with the attempt to mix-n-match traits. Examples of this include taking the gene of a spider and inserting it into the DNA of a goat so we could milk the goat to get spider web protein to make bulletproof vests; or taking human genes and inserting it in corn to make spermicide. It's messing with Mother Nature—big mistake!

The GMO's currently in our diet have bacterial or viral genes that are inserted into the following crops:

1. Soy
2. Corn (including high fructose corn syrup, corn oil, corn syrup)
3. Sugar Beets (most sugar is the U.S.)
4. Canola (as in canola oil)
5. Cotton (including cottonseed oil)
6. Alfalfa
7. Zucchini and yellow squash
8. Papaya (from China and Hawaii)

Note: Popcorn is a type of corn (Zea mays everta) that is not GMO. It is however heavily covered in pesticides, insecticides, herbicides, fungicides, and fertilizers, and that means that it's best to buy organic.

With almost ninety percent of commercial crops being genetically engineered in the United States (corn, soy and sugar are the biggest), it's become a huge problem for everyone, especially our developing children. The biotech industry wants to genetically engineer the rest of the food supply too including the livestock and fish. This is irreversible and in my opinion very dangerous. There are two (soon to be three) modifications to corn crops that everyone needs to know—Bt-toxin, glyphosate resistance, and 2,4-D (the most recently approved pesticide) resistance.

The first, and perhaps the most disturbing, is that corn (that summertime cookout classic) has been engineered with a gene from bacterium called Bt, which allows the corn to synthesize a toxin that blows up the stomach of an insect. This potent toxin can't be washed off—it's part of the genetic makeup of the GMO corn. This sure sounds like a potential risk for leaky gut to me.

The second modification on corn is the gene that allows the crop to thrive in the presence of glyphosate. Glyphosate (the herbicide found in commercial brand Roundup) is a chemical that kills weeds and plants. Therefore, by modifying the genes of the crop, the crop is afforded protection against the chemical treatment. Monsanto, the company that manufactures Roundup, is the same company who manufactures the GMO seeds that withstand this toxic herbicide—this is known as "Roundup Ready" crops. Prior to Roundup Ready crops, Roundup was typically applied before planting to kill weeds. Because the crop species were sensitive to roundup, the herbicide could not be generally applied after the crop species started to grow. The use of GMO seeds/plants allows for applications of Roundup during the growth of the crops has turned out to be the solution for controlling weed growth. But at what cost to human health?

You might also be interested to know that glyphosate is patented as a microbicide—essentially, it's an antibiotic. We know that chronic low doses of antibiotics lead to antibiotic resistance in microbes. Perhaps this explains why we are faced with hospital infections that are unresponsive to antibiotic treatment.

And finally, possibly coming soon to a market near you, is a corn crop that is resistant to 2,4-D. This chemical 2,4-Dichlorophenoxyacetic acid (2,4-D), once made up half of the herbicide mix known as Agent Orange. Risks to eating corn with 2,4-D resistance could include skin sores, liver damage and death in animals. 2,4-D is a potential endocrine disruptor and can affect development. Rats exposed to 2,4-D exhibited depressed thyroid hormone levels, which can affect normal metabolism and brain functioning. Studies found that men who were exposed to 2,4-D had lower sperm counts and more sperm abnormalities than those unexposed to the herbicide.

Similar to what we are witnessing with antibiotic resistance bacteria in humans as a result of overuse of antibiotic prescriptions in health care and antibiotic use in factory-farmed livestock, we can see a similar trend in herbicide-resistance crops. In the past 15 years since herbicide-resistant crops were first introduced, weeds already have become resistant to herbicides affiliated with genetically engineered crops. Monsanto's Roundup has led to glyphosate-resistant weeds, a problem that is driving farmers to apply older, more toxic herbicides and to reduce conservation tilling to combat weeds. Now, to treat the problem of glyphosate-resistant weeds, biotech companies are simply creating crops resistant to a variety of chemicals. It's only a matter of time before we are eating more and more chemicals in every bite.

We have yet to fully comprehend the health risk of eating GMOs, but many researchers have provided some insight into the potential harm to humans by boldly stating "They cause disease." In an interview by consumer advocate Jeffrey Smith with Dr. Stephanie Seneff, a research scientist at the Massachusetts Institute of Technology (MIT), glyphosate was identifies as possibly "the most important factor in the development of multiple chronic diseases and conditions that have become prevalent in Westernized societies," including, but not limited to:

- Autism
- Allergies
- Cancer
- Parkinson's disease
- IBS, Chronic diarrhea, Chron's disease, Colitis

- Obesity
- Depression
- Cardiovascular disease
- Infertility
- Alzheimer's disease
- Multiple Sclerosis[45]

According to Dr. Senneff, the Bt toxin which kills insects by destroying the cell walls of their digestive track is not specific to insects and has been shown to poke holes in human cells, damaging the intestines and causing leaky gut. A peer-reviewed report authored by Anthony Samsel, a retired science consultant and Dr. Stephanie Seneff, reveals how glyphosate wrecks human health.

While Monsanto insists that Roundup is safe for humans, Seneff and Samsel's research tells a different story altogether. Their report, published in the journal *Entropy* argues that glyphosate residues, found in most commonly consumed foods in the Western diet courtesy of GE sugar, corn, soy and wheat, "enhance the damaging effects of other food-borne chemical residues and toxins in the environment to disrupt normal body functions and induce disease."[46] Interestingly, your gut bacteria are a key component of glyphosate's mechanism of harm.

Monsanto claims that Roundup is harmless to animals and humans because the mechanism of action it uses (which allows it to kill weeds), called the shikimate pathway, is absent in all animals. However, the shikimate pathway *is* present in our gut bacteria, and that's the key to understanding how it causes such widespread systemic harm in both humans and animals.

The bacteria in your body outnumber your cells by ten to one. For every cell in your body, you have ten microbes of various kinds, and all of them have the shikimate pathway, so they will *all* respond to the presence of glyphosate! Glyphosate causes extreme disruption of the microbe's function and lifecycle. What's worse, glyphosate *preferentially* affects *beneficial* bacteria, allowing pathogens to overgrow and take over.[47] At that point, your body also has to contend with the toxins produced by the pathogens. Once the chronic inflammation sets in, you're well on your way toward chronic and potentially debilitating disease.

A study republished in 2014 showed that rats on a diet of GMO corn suffered increased tumor growth and early mortality when compared to a control group[48]. GMOs have been correlated with a long list of health problems, including thyroid cancer, kidney disease, rheumatoid arthritis, and infertility. Once thought to be protected in the womb, even our babies are at risk before they ever eat their first meal. Research from Canada shows a Bt toxin (Cry1Ab protein) in pregnant women and their fetuses.[49]

One fact worth noting is the dramatic rise in people with multiple chronic diseases, allergies, celiac disease and non-celiac gluten sensitivity since GMOs were introduced in the United States in 1996. The graph below shows the increase in deaths due to intestinal infection and the application of glyphosate to wheat.

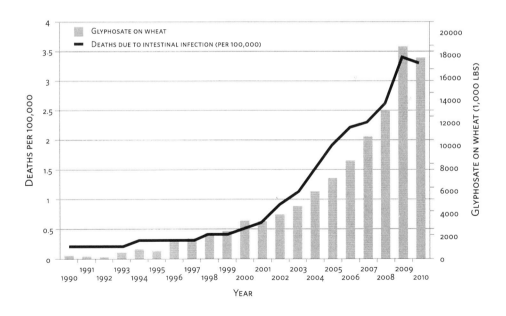

Source: Samsel and Seneff (2013)

Could there be a connection between the epidemic of gluten intolerance and the increased use of Monsanto's glyphosate herbicide Roundup? According to a compelling peer-reviewed report from two U.S. scientists Samsel and Seneff, this is highly possible. Farmers are now using glyphosate not only to control weeds but also to dry down wheat, rice, sugarcane and other crops just before harvest; resulting in higher residues in the foods we eat. The following abstract from the paper *"Glyphosate, Pathways to Modern Diseases II: Celiac Sprue and Gluten Intolerance"*[50] proposes the connection between the increased use of glyphosate with growing rates of celiac incidence, deaths from intestinal infections, acute kidney disease and deaths due to Parkinson's disease.

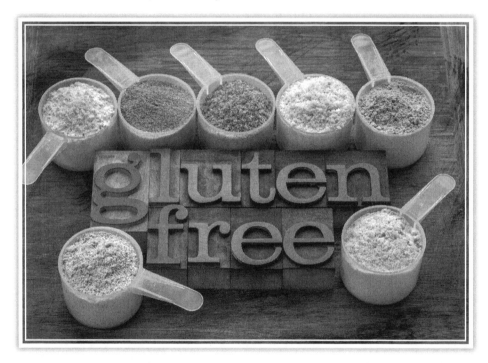

ABSTRACT:

Celiac disease, and more generally, gluten intolerance, is a growing problem worldwide, but especially in North America and Europe, where an estimated 5 percent of the population now suffers from it. **Symptoms include nausea, diarrhea, skin rashes, macrocytic anemia and depression. It is a multifactorial disease associated with numerous nutritional deficiencies as well as reproductive issues and increased risk to thyroid disease, kidney failure and cancer.** Here, we propose that glyphosate, the active ingredient in the herbicide, Roundup, is the most important causal factor of this epidemic. **Fish exposed to glyphosate develop digestive problems that are reminiscent of celiac disease. Celiac disease is associated with imbalances of gut bacteria that can be fully explained by the known effects of glyphosate on gut bacteria.** Characteristics of celiac disease point to impairment in many cytochrome P450 enzymes, which are involved with detoxifying environmental toxins, activating vitamin D3, catabolizing vitamin A, and maintaining bile acid production and sulfate supplies to the gut. Glyphosate is known to inhibit cytochrome P450 enzymes. Deficiencies in iron, cobalt, molybdenum, copper and other rare metals associated with celiac disease can be attributed to glyphosate's strong ability to chelate these elements. Deficiencies in tryptophan, tyrosine, methionine, and selenomethionine associated with celiac disease match glyphosate's known depletion of these amino acids. **Celiac disease patients have an increased risk to non-Hodgkin's lymphoma, which has been implicated in glyphosate exposure. Glyphosate residues in wheat and other crops are likely increasing recently due to the growing practice of crop desiccation just prior to harvest.** We argue that the practice of "ripening" sugar cane with glyphosate may explain the recent surge in kidney failure among agricultural workers in Central America. We conclude with a plea to governments to reconsider policies regarding the safety of glyphosate residues in foods.

This chart shows the increased rate of hospital discharge diagnosis of celiac disease in correlation to the increased application of glyphosate to wheat.[51]

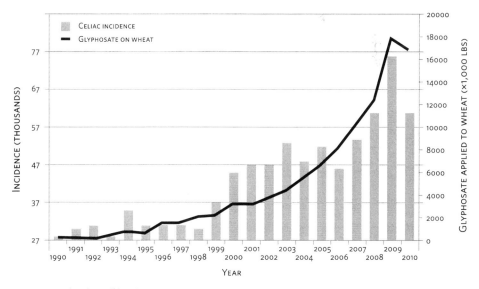

Source: Samsel and Seneff (2013)

For the past thirty years, Dr. Seneff has been passionate about finding out potential causes of autism, after her friend's son was diagnosed. She points out the correlations between increased glyphosate use over recent years and dramatic increase in autism rates. It's no surprise that finding a potential cause of autism is a topic that I am deeply interested in. Personally, I don't think it is any one thing. In fact, I think we miss the point when we try to blame any one issue or spend all our energy searching for a cure. Instead, we need to focus our attention on the common thread that runs through each case of autism and begin to piece together what we can do to prevent autism. I think this connection to GMO's and glyphosate is worth exploring in great detail.

We know the rate of autism has risen dramatically. In fact the latest statistics by the CDC show that one in fifty children in the U.S. now fall within the autism spectrum with a 5:1 boy to girl ratio. This represents a twenty-three percent increase since 2010 and a seventy-eight percent increase since 2007. I'm sure we all remember when the incidence of autism in the U.S. was one in ten thousand. This is not a case of improved diagnostic tools; It's an epidemic!

So, it begs the question—what has changed? Our environment and our food!

Dr. Seneff identified two key problems in autism that are unrelated to the brain yet clearly associated with the condition that I think I worth pointing out. They are both linked with glyphosate exposure:

1. Gut dysbiosis (imbalances in gut bacteria, inflammation, leaky gut, food allergies such as gluten intolerance)

2. Disrupted sulfur metabolism / sulfur and sulfate deficiency

Interestingly, certain microbes in your body actually break down glyphosate, which is a good thing. However, a byproduct of this action is ammonia, and children with autism tend to have significantly higher levels of ammonia in their blood than the general population.[52] This is true for Alzheimer's disease as well. In your brain, ammonia causes encephalitis (brain inflammation).

Another devastating agent you really do not want in your body is formaldehyde, which a recent nutritional analysis discovered is present in genetically engineered corn at a level that is two hundred *times* the amount that animal studies have determined to be toxic to animals. Formaldehyde destroys DNA.

When it comes to considering the glyphosate-autism connection, Dr. Seneff is not alone. Former U.S. Navy staff scientist Dr. Nancy Swanson, who holds a Ph.D. in physics, five U.S. patents and has authored more than thirty scientific papers, agrees. Ten years ago, she became seriously ill, and in her journey to regain her health she turned to organic foods. Not surprisingly her symptoms dramatically improved. She has meticulously collected statistics on glyphosate usage and various diseases and conditions, including autism.

GMOs CROSS-CONTAMINATE NON-GMO CROPS

Soon it will be difficult to find any crops unaffected. Farmers can't protect against cross-pollination by wind and insects, and the resulting seed will be a hybrid of their non-GMO crop with the GMO crop. Corn is one of the most commonly genetically engineered foods, with about ninety percent of it being GMO, and due to cross-pollination, that remaining ten percent is not guaranteed to be GMO-free for long.

PROTECT YOURSELF AND YOUR FAMILY

It's important to understand that the glyphosate sprayed on conventional and genetically engineered crops actually becomes systemic throughout the plant, so it cannot be washed off. It's *inside* the plant. For example, genetically engineered corn has been found to contain 13 ppm of glyphosate, compared to zero in non-GMO corn. At *13 ppm*, GMO corn contains more than *eighteen times* the "safe" level of glyphosate set by the Environmental Protection Agency (EPA). Organ damage in animals has occurred at levels as low as 0.1 ppm.

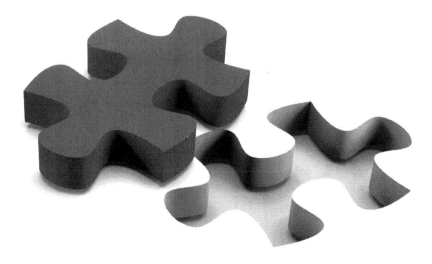

Foods labeled 100% USDA organic cannot lawfully contain GMOs. Buying one hundred percent organic ensures not only that your food is non-GMO, but also free from dangerous pesticides, hormones, and other chemicals. Look for labels that say "100% Organic" or "USDA Organic." Assume that anything labeled "Made With Organic" contains some organic ingredients, and the rest may be GMO. Read labels carefully until you find the brands you trust.

THE "DIRTY DOZEN"

If you're on a budget and need to prioritize your organic purchases, or you would simply like to know which type of produce has the highest pesticide residues—and which do not.

12 MOST CONTAMINATED	12 LEAST CONTAMINATED
1. Peaches	1. Onions
2. Apples	2. Avocado
3. Sweet Bell Peppers	3. Sweet Corn (Frozen)
4. Celery	4. Pineapples
5. Nectarines	5. Mango
6. Strawberries	6. Asparagus
7. Cherries	7. Sweet Peas (Frozen)
8. Pears	8. Kiwi Fruit
9. Grapes (Imported)	9. Bananas
10. Spinach	10. Cabbage
11. Lettuce	11. Broccoli
12. Potatoes	12. Papaya

Source: Environmental Working Group, www.ewg.org and Food News, www.foodnews.org

QUALITY OVER QUANTITY: MEAT AND DAIRY

When cows are fed inflammatory GMO crops like corn and soy, they become sick. Cows were meant to graze in natural sunlight eating grass. If you include meat and dairy in your diet, choose organic, grass-fed products.

LOOK FOR NON-GMO PROJECT VERIFIED PRODUCTS

The Non-GMO Project is an independent organization that verifies foods that do not contain any genetically engineered ingredients. They are the only such organization in the U.S. and Canada. Keep in mind that food manufacturers are getting savvy on tricking the consumer. Some will claim to avoid GMO ingredients, but they are not Non-GMO certified because the dairy they use comes from cows being fed GMO corn and soy.

The non-GMO movement is gaining momentum thanks to social media and the work of organizations like the Institute for Responsible Technology (IRT). They have made it their mission to research the effects of GMOs and educate the public and the government. One of the biggest things you can do is boycott GMO products.

Avoid using Roundup weed killer around your home where children and pets can come into contact with it simply by playing in the yard.

To learn more about this important topic and the risks associated with GMO's watch the film *Genetic Roulette: The Gamble of Our Lives.* You deserve to know exactly what you're putting in your body.

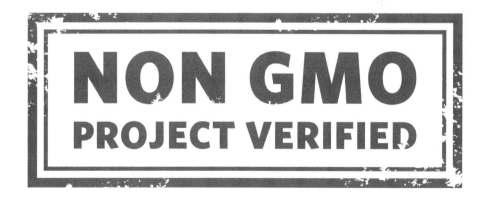

ENVIRONMENTAL TRIGGERS:
COUNTING CHEMICALS, NOT CALORIES

Now that you're informed about the foods that may be triggering an immune response like gluten, MSG and GMOS's, you should also keep in mind the thousands of different herbicides and pesticides that are applied to conventionally grown foods. But beyond our food supply, environmental triggers also impact your health in dramatic ways that you should know.

Today's conveniences have come at a price. You can't see, smell, taste or feel the toxins in our food, water or air and yet it's estimated that Americans have between four hundred to eight hundred chemicals stored in their body. I believe one of the main reasons people experience weight loss resistance is due to chemical toxicity. We know that toxins are stored in the adipose (fat) tissue. Your body is protecting you from the toxins by holding on to the fat. So to lose weight, you would need to safely detoxify the body first.

Chemicals from your environment often have the ability to interfere with your delicate hormonal system and can have a huge impact on how your body functions, especially metabolism and hormones. Even very small amounts can lead to weight gain, neurological problems, reproductive problems, skin conditions and more. There are chemicals today in the U.S. that have been banned for years but are still present in our environment mostly because they are resistant to breaking down. An example of this are PCBs, which are linked to damaging the brain development of babies still in the womb, various types of cancers, and hormone disruption. One of the places PCBs can be found is in farm-raised salmon because they are fed ground-up fish and fish oils that have absorbed higher levels of the chemical.

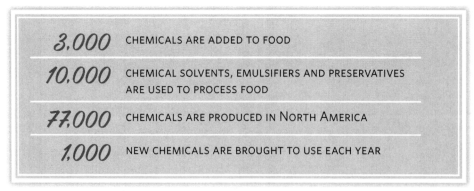

3,000	CHEMICALS ARE ADDED TO FOOD
10,000	CHEMICAL SOLVENTS, EMULSIFIERS AND PRESERVATIVES ARE USED TO PROCESS FOOD
77,000	CHEMICALS ARE PRODUCED IN NORTH AMERICA
1,000	NEW CHEMICALS ARE BROUGHT TO USE EACH YEAR

Let's discuss some of the most prevalent environmental triggers lurking in your home and how to avoid them.

Bisphenol-A (BPA)

Bisphenol-A (BPA) is one of the most pervasive chemicals on the market today. It is used to make clear, unbreakable plastic everyday products like sippy cups, storage containers, and toys. It is also used as an epoxy-film to line the inside of all kinds of canned foods and baby formula and is found on cash register receipt paper. Sadly, it's almost impossible to avoid these days with over six billion pounds being produced annually, much of which ends up in thousands of consumer products. In fact, ninety-three percent of Americans have detectable levels of BPA in their bodies, according to the U.S. Centers for Disease Control and Prevention.[53]

Inside the body, BPA acts as an estrogen mimic, interfering with our sensitive endocrine system and affecting fetal development during pregnancy, increasing your risk of breast cancer and interfering with age of puberty in young girls. It has been linked to type-2 diabetes, obesity, and attention deficit hyperactivity disorder (ADHD) in children. Even tiny amounts of BPA can trigger changes in the body that lead to serious health problems.

How to Avoid BPA

- Choose fresh or frozen foods instead of canned. A 2011 study showed that people decreased the amount of BPA in their bodies by sixty percent in just three days when they eliminated canned foods and food packaged in plastics from their diet.[54] Another study found that eating one can of soup every day for five days increased the BPA in your body by twelve hundred percent![55]

- If you do buy canned food, buy from the few canned food companies now using BPA-free can liners. Some options include, Eden Organics, Westbrae Natural, Hunt's, Healthy Choice, and HJ Heinz.

- Skip the plastic food containers. Use glass or stainless steel.

- Store food in glass or ceramic containers.

- Decline your receipts when you can. BPA rubs off easily onto hands, and then gets into mouths or eyes. Store receipts you need in an envelope separate from your wallet or purse, and wash your hands after handling them.

A special note about "BPA-free" plastics. Researchers have tested thirty-five toddler drinking cups labeled "BPA-free" at two independent labs. The results showed nine of the sippy cups had significant amounts of estrogen-like activity, while seven of those cups had higher activity levels than those made with BPA.

According to Lara Adler, an expert in exposure routes and impacts of environmental chemicals, many of the manufacturers of BPA-Free products simply swapped out Bisphenol-A with a similar chemical in the Bisphenol family, namely BPS. She says that newer studies into BPS have found it to have a similar, if not more powerful impact on our bodies than BPA. In this regard, she feels that BPA-free claims often amount to a marketing gimmick!

In my opinion, it's not worth the risk. There's so much we don't know about the safety of these chemicals and I'm not willing to risk giving them to my children. Glass and stainless steel are easy to find and safe.

Triclosan

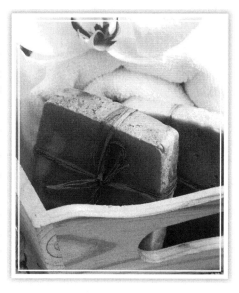

Triclosan is a man-made synthetic antimicrobial chemical designed to kill germs. Yet it doesn't kill viruses, which are the causes of colds and the flu. It's commonly found in antibacterial soaps and hand sanitizers, tarter control toothpaste, and some deodorants and fragrances. Exposure to triclosan has been associated with hormone disruption and increased risk of breast cancer. It's been found in blood and in breast milk. It's also bioaccumulative so it builds up in your body and it doesn't break down easily.

Some believe the overuse of antibacterial soaps and disinfectant products has led to the creation of resistant bacteria and viruses leaving us with fewer tools to fight infectious diseases.

When it's washed off skin and down the drain, it also ends up in our lakes, rivers, and other water supplies, where it's toxic to aquatic life. It even ends up in sludge that's applied to agricultural lands as a fertilizer, contaminating that soil as well.

The bottom line is that the use of triclosan is unnecessary. Studies have shown that this toxic chemical is **no more effective** at preventing illness or removing germs than soap and water.

PBDEs

Polybrominated diphenyl ethers (PBDEs) are a class of flame retardant chemicals used to make household objects less likely to catch fire like polyurethane foam found in upholstered furniture and bedding, computers and other electronics. They shed off of these products and build up in household dust and indoor air. Once they are in the dust in your home, they enter your body through your respiratory system. Children and pets have much higher levels of PBDE's in their bodies because of crawling around on the floor and being close to the house dust that accumulates there. Some studies have found that children can have more than three times the levels in their blood than adults.[56]

Because these chemicals are bioaccumulative, they are able to build up in your body and don't break down easily, making them difficult to remove. Exposure has been linked to hormone disruption, thyroid problems, and reproductive harm like undescended testicles, delayed puberty, reduced fertility, low birth weight, and birth defects. Exposure to PBDEs in the womb is associated with lower IQs.

They've been detected in breast milk, which is particularly concerning because developing children, infants, and fetuses are at highest risk to PBDEs.

Twelve states and the European Union have banned certain PBDEs, but the U.S. government as a whole has not taken action on these toxic chemicals. Studies have shown that American adults have ten to one hundred times higher levels of PBDEs in their bodies than adults in other countries, and the highest human levels in the world tested to date have been found in pregnant women in California.

How to Avoid PBDEs

Reduce exposure to house dust by cleaning your home with a wet mop or by using a vacuum with a HEPA filter. Remove your shoes at the door to avoid tracking chemicals inside and wash your hands throughout the day with soap and water, which has been shown to reduce PBDE levels in your blood significantly.

....

Note about electronics and products: Certain PBDE-free products are now available from Canon, Dell, HP, Intel, Erickson, Apple, Acer, Nokia, Motorola, LG Electronics, and Sony.

Parabens

Parabens are used to prevent the growth of microbes in cosmetic products but they can be absorbed through our skin. Parabens are founds in a wide variety of products like shampoos, conditioners, facial and body cleaners, lotions, deodorants, and eye makeup. They are found in higher concentrations in products that are more liquid, like shampoos and body lotions.

Parabans are a *class* of chemicals (there are six different types commonly found in personal care products) and have been found in nearly every urine sample tested of the U.S. adult population.[57] They have even been found in the biopsies from breast tumors.[58] Parabens mimic estrogen by binding to estrogen receptors on cells. They also increase expression of genes normally regulated by a natural form of estrogen (estradiol). These genes cause breast cancer cells to multiply and grow according to cellular studies.[59] Health risks include reproductive toxicity, allergies, skin irritation, neurotoxicity and immune issues. The most vulnerable population includes pregnant women and children.

Its label name:

Ethylparaben, butylparaben, methylparaben, propylparaben, other ingredients ending in—*paraben*

How to avoid:

Look for "paraben-free" products. Search the Skin Deep Database for brands that avoid parabens.

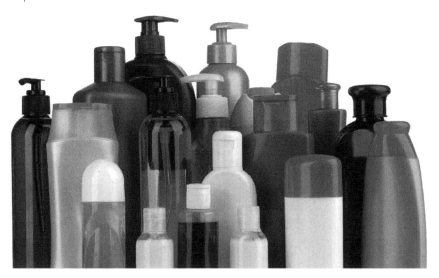

Phthalates

Phthalates are used to soften plastics and extend the life of fragrance. If you recall the smell of a new vinyl shower curtain—that's phthalates. They are also used in air fresheners, perfumes, detergents, cleaning products, nail polish and cosmetics.

Its label name:

phthalate, DEP, DBP, fragrance, perfume, parfum

In a 2002 report titled "Not Too Pretty," phthalates where detected in nearly three-fourths of tested products, even though none of the seventy-two products had phthalates listed on the labels.[60] Follow-up testing conducted by the Campaign in 2008 found that some of the products tested in 2002 contained lower levels of phthalates. A significant loophole in federal law allows phthalates (and other chemicals) to be added to fragrances without disclosure to consumers.

Diethyl phthalate, DEP, is frequently used in fragrance, but it is rarely if ever listed on ingredient labels. An extensive study of twenty-five hundred individuals found metabolites of at least one phthalate in ninety-seven percent of the tested group[61].

Research suggests that phthalates are endocrine disrupters, which can cause harm during critical periods of development. Phthalate exposure in pregnant women has been associated with a shortened distance between the anus and genitals in their male babies, indicating a feminization had occurred during prenatal genital development.[62] Phthalates are also associated with poor sperm count in men, infertility, small testicles, and low levels of sex hormones.

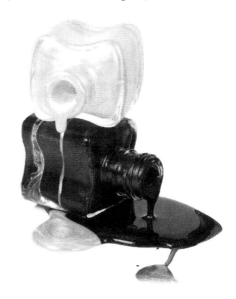

How to avoid:

Look for labels that indicate "phthalate-free." Products that list "fragrance" on the label should be avoided to prevent possible exposure to phthalates.

Wearing and Breathing Poison

If you use fabric softener, you are coating your towels, sheets and clothes with toxic chemicals. They are being absorbed through your skin and your lungs. Here is a snapshot of what you are wearing:

- CHLOROFORM: A carcinogenic neurotoxin listed in the EPA's Hazardous Waste list. Inhaling its vapors may cause loss of consciousness, nausea, headache, vomiting, and/or dizziness, drowsiness. It may aggravate disorders of the heart, kidneys or liver. Its effects worsen when subjected to heat.

- A-TERPINEOL: Causes Central Nervous System (CNS) disorders, meaning problems relating to the brain and spine such as Alzheimer's disease, ADD, dementia, Multiple Sclerosis, Parkinson's disease, seizures, strokes, and Sudden Infant Death Syndrome. Early symptoms of CNS problems include aphasia, blurred vision, disorientation, dizziness, headaches, hunger, memory loss, numbness in face, pain in neck and spine. It also irritates the mucous membranes and, if you breathe it in, can cause respiratory depression, pneumonia ,or fatal edema.

- BENZYL ALCOHOL: This upper respiratory tract irritant can cause central nervous system (CNS) disorders, headache, nausea, vomiting, dizziness, and dramatic drops in blood pressure.

- BENZYL ACETATE: This substances has been linked to pancreatic cancer. Its vapors can be irritating to eyes and respiratory passages and it can also be absorbed through the skin.

- ETHANOL: This ingredient, which is also on the EPA's Hazardous Waste list, and linked to CNS disorders.

- PENTANE: A chemical known to be harmful if inhaled.

- ETHYL ACETATE: This substance, which is on the EPA's Hazardous Waste list, can be irritating to the eyes and respiratory tract. It may also cause severe headaches and loss of consciousness, as well as damage to the liver and kidneys.

- CAMPHOR: Another substance on the EPA's Hazardous Waste list. It is easily absorbed through body tissue, causing irritation of eyes, nose and throat. Camphor can also cause dizziness, confusion, nausea, twitching muscles and convulsions.

- LINALOOL: A narcotic known to cause respiratory problems and CNS disorders. In animal testing, exposure to linalool has resulted in death.

- **PHTHALATES:** Used in scented products to help the scent last longer, phthalates have been linked to breast cancer and reproductive system problems.

- **LIMONENE:** This known carcinogen can cause irritation to eyes and skin.[63]

With so much to think about it can feel overwhelming to think about environmental triggers as yet another contributor of disease. But consider this, the number of chemicals on the market today is breathtaking (literally). And the number of children in the U.S. with one or more developmental disabilities, from a subtle learning disability to overt behavioral or emotional disorders, is on the rise. We know, exposure to environmental toxins have been linked with higher rates of mental retardation, intellectual impairment, and behavioral problems, such as conduct disorder and attention deficit hyperactivity disorder.[64] This can't be overlooked as a potential trigger for all health issues. Don't you agree? Reducing your exposure is an important step to improving your quality of life.

Here is how I took control and evaluated the safety of the chemicals in my environment. Simply visit the Skin Deep Database from the Environmental Working Group at http://www.ewg.org/skindeep/. There are almost seventy thousand products in the database. They use a rating scale of 0 to 2 low hazard; 3 to 6 moderate hazard; and 7 to 10 high hazard. They also provide a scale on ingredients concerns in the areas of cancer, developmental and reproductive toxicity, allergies and immune-toxicity. You can put the name of the products you use everyday. I decided anything with a rating of five or above got tossed immediately. Then I started replacing products that were rated in the moderate zone with the goal of using all products in the low hazard. In many instances, I realized we didn't need some of the products we had become accustomed too. For example, we completely eliminated the use of fabric softener, mouthwash, body lotions, hand sanitizers, air fresheners, perfume, and more.

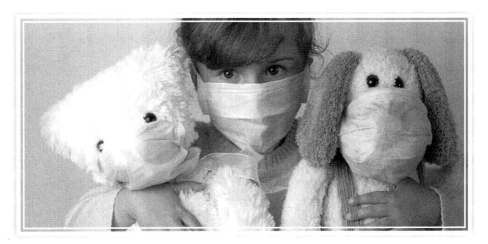

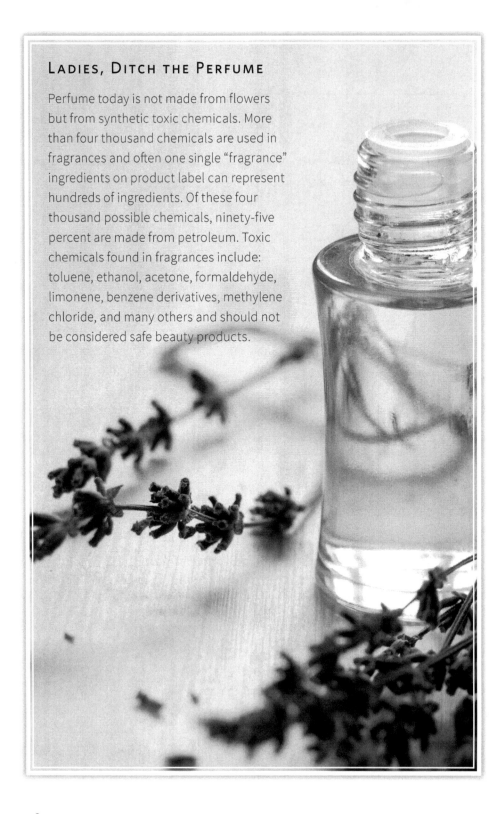

LADIES, DITCH THE PERFUME

Perfume today is not made from flowers but from synthetic toxic chemicals. More than four thousand chemicals are used in fragrances and often one single "fragrance" ingredients on product label can represent hundreds of ingredients. Of these four thousand possible chemicals, ninety-five percent are made from petroleum. Toxic chemicals found in fragrances include: toluene, ethanol, acetone, formaldehyde, limonene, benzene derivatives, methylene chloride, and many others and should not be considered safe beauty products.

15 Toxic Trespassers

HARMFUL CHEMICALS TO AVOID IN PRODUCTS WOMEN USE EVERYDAY

CHEMICAL	PRODUCTS IT LURKS IN	POTENTIAL HEALTH PROBLEMS	AVOIDING IT
1,4-dioxane No More Toxic Tub	Products that create suds, like shampoo, liquid soap, bubble bath, hair relaxers	Cancer Birth defects	Read labels to avoid chemicals that may signal the presence of 1,4-dioxane, like sodium laureth sulfate, PEG, "ceteareth", and "oleth".
2-butoxyethanol Household Hazards	Glass cleaners, all-purpose spray cleaners	Reduced fertility low birth weight	Make your own non-toxic cleaners with WVE's recipes, or buy from the few companies that disclose all ingredients on the label and look to avoid it.
Alkyl phenol ethoxylates (APEs) Household Hazards	Laundry detergents, stain removers, and all-purpose cleaners	Reproductive harm	Make your own non-toxic cleaners with WVE's recipes, or buy from the few companies that disclose all ingredients on the label and look to avoid it.
Ammonium quaternary compounds Disinfectant Overkill	Some disinfectant sprays, toilet cleaners, alcohol-free hand sanitizers	Occupational asthma Decreased fertility and birth defects	Reduce your use of disinfectant products; download WVE's Reduce Your Use of Disinfectants fact sheet for ideas.
Bisphenol-A (BPA) No Silver Lining	Plastics like baby bottles, sippy cups, water bottles, and children's toys; can linings	Breast cancer early puberty Hormone disruption	Opt for fresh or frozen foods instead of canned, look for plastics labeled "BPA-free" and never microwave plastic.
Formaldehyde Glossed Over The Blowup on Blowouts	Some nail products, shampoos, body washes, chemical hair straighteners	Cancer Skin and respiratory irritation	Look for nail polishes and hardeners labeled "three- free" or "formaldehyde-free" and avoid chemical hair straighteners.
Hydroquinone Toxic Products Marketed to Black Women	Skin lighteners	Cancer Immune system damage Reproductive/ developmental harm	Avoid skin lighteners with hydroquinone listed on the label.
Lead A Poison Kiss & Pretty Scary	Some lipsticks and other cosmetics, sunscreens, whitening toothpastes, children's face paint	Reproductive / developmental harm Nerve, joint, and muscle disorders Heart, bone, and kidney problems	Contact the company and ask if lead is a contaminant in the product.

Monoethanolamine (MEA) Household Hazards	Some laundry detergents, all-purpose cleaners and floor cleaners	Occupational asthma	Make your own cleaners with WVE's recipes or buy from the few companies that disclose all ingredients on the label and look to avoid it.
PBDEs (Flame retardants) Flame Retardants in Baby Products	Polyurethane foam padding in furniture, children's products	Reproductive / developmental harm Thyroid hormone disruption	Avoid products containing polyurethane foam which indicate "TB117 compliant" on the label. Look for products stuffed with cotton, polyester or wool instead of foam.
Phthalates Glossed Over What's That Smell? Not So Sexy	Fragrances in cleaning products, personal care products, cosmetics & nail polish	Reduced fertility Increased risk of breast cancer Genital malformations in baby boys Increased allergic symptoms and asthma in children	Avoid products with synthetic fragrance; look for fragrance with essential oils or products labeled "fragrance-free." Look for nail polishes labeled "three-free" or "phthalate-free."
Sodium laureth sulfate No More Toxic Tub	Soaps, shampoos, toothpaste, and products that create suds	Products containing these chemicals may contain 1,4-dioxane (see above)	Read labels to avoid products containing sodium laureth sulfate.
Synthetic musks: galaxolide and tonalide What's That Smell?	Fragrances, such as in cleaning products and personal care products	Hormone disruption Breakdown of the body's defenses against other toxic exposures Increased risk of breast cancer	Avoid products with synthetic fragrance; look for fragrance with essential oils or products labeled "fragrance-free."
Toluene Glossed Over	Nail salon products	Headache, dizziness, fatigue Eyes, nose & throat irritation Reproductive/ developmental harm	Look for nail polishes labeled "three-free" or "toluene-free."
Triclosan Disinfectant Overkill	Antibacterial hand & dish soaps, some disinfectant products, tartar-control toothpastes, fragrance	Hormone disruption Potential increased risk of breast cancer	Avoid antibacterial hand soap, and read labels to avoid products containing triclosan as an active ingredient.

*We do not intend to imply that use of products containing these chemicals has been proven to cause these health effects. In most cases, the research to prove the safety of use of these products has never been conducted. Rather, we believe that from a precautionary standpoint, the presence of these chemicals in products we use everyday poses an unnecessary potential risk which can be avoided.

Source: Women's Voices for the Earth

Part II: Education Takeaways

What you eat is important, but what you digest is even more important. Proper digestion is the foundation of health.

Understanding the basic functions of the human body is critical to your success. Find a health coach or practitioner who is willing to teach you and listen to you.

Each system of the body is interconnected.
Health conditions affecting one system
will impact all the others.
You must treat the whole body not the individual parts.

Digestive and hormonal issues are very common and require support, diet and lifestyle changes. Get functional lab tests and explore ways to care for yourself on a deeper level.

Learn what foods and lifestyle behaviors are feeding your disease. Dietary triggers like gluten, genetically modified foods, additives and soy can be triggering an immune response in the body leading to disease. Food sensitivities and conditions like non-celiac gluten sensitivity should be taken very seriously. Your life depends on it.

Consider environmental toxins as a potential immune system trigger and reduce your overall toxin burden.

Ask yourself today:

Is my body functioning well?

What foods and lifestyle behaviors are feeding my disease?

What products do I use everyday
that could be negatively affecting my health?
(Visit www.ewg.org to check the safety.)

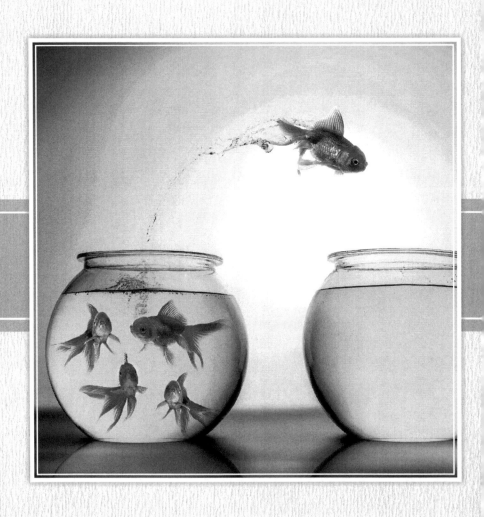

PART III: Action

Building a Foundation

This is where you learn to take back your power. The health of your gut is central to your entire health. In fact, it is connected to everything that happens in your body. Everything! You can build the foundation of your health by becoming your own nutrition detective and implementing the key steps to rebuild digestive health.

THE ELIMINATION DIET

Removing all food sensitivities is a critical step in the process of restoring your health or getting a baseline for what your body feels like when it is not in an inflamed state. This step is often more of a refinement of your diet, before determining what your typical diet will be going forward. However, many times a person's main issues stem from food sensitivities and therefore the removal of the offending foods may be the only changes needed.

THE MAIN AREAS AFFECTED ARE:

- Digestion
- Elimination
- Inflammation and pain
- Mood and energy

This diet (also known as the "testing diet") requires a **strict** elimination of the possible problematic ingredients for ten days, including:

- Gluten (all forms)
- Dairy
- Eggs
- Corn
- Peanuts
- Soy
- Food colorings (Yellow #6, Red #40, etc.), food additives, and preservatives.

Also—lower or remove sugar. The reason sugar is listed here is that sweet and starchy foods raise blood sugar, which raise insulin, which lead to inflammation. For sweetness, include natural sugars in small amounts, like raw honey, pure maple syrup, dates, etc.

Remove: Artificial sweeteners. In addition to being neuroexcititory (i.e. making it difficult to sleep and creating anxiety), artificial sweeteners like aspartame, Splenda (sucralose), Sweet-N-Low, and high fructose corn syrup disrupt healthy gut flora, allowing bad bacteria to take over. They can lead to serious digestive problems too.

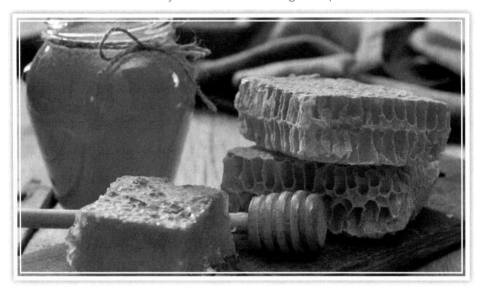

Reintroduction

Introduce one food back at a time is introduced into the diet by ingesting two servings—one serving for breakfast and one serving for lunch starting on day eleven. By the end of the day, at least a typical amount of the food has been eaten. Record the results over the course of three days. If you don't experience any of the symptoms on the checklist (i.e. the food is not offending) you may continue to include that food in our daily diet. A new food is introduced ("tested") every **three** days and you will record the results again for each one before introducing the next food. It takes approximately one month to complete the elimination/testing diet.

Please be honest with yourself during an elimination diet. This is your chance to be a health detective and it's worth doing it correctly. I can't tell you how many people have told me they had "no issues" with a particular food only to find out after further questioning that symptoms did show up. Cheese seems to be the number one food that falls into the "I feel fine, except for a little stuffiness and maybe some constipation" category.

....

Note: The reintroduction of colorings, additives, preservatives and artificial sweeteners is not recommended.

1. Corn (must be organic or non-GMO certified)

2. Peanuts (unless you have a known allergy to peanuts or mold)

3. Eggs (preferably free-range, organic)

4. Soy (fermented soy like natto, tempeh, miso. Skip if you don't enjoy these foods)

5. Dairy (ideally, raw, non-pasteurized)

6. Gluten (unless an autoimmune condition is present)

An elimination diet is not a lifestyle diet. It is short-term and only intended to help you identify food sensitivities. It need not feel restrictive. Typically you would include a variety of hypoallergenic foods like, meat, fish, poultry, fruit, vegetables, rice, legumes (except peanuts), nuts and seeds, and non-gluten grains, like millet, quinoa, and amaranth. Once the body has adjusted to the absence of suspected foods, those foods are systematically added back into the diet, and any resulting symptoms are recorded. An elimination diet, when carefully planned, provides sufficient amounts of all essential nutrients.

Individuals following an elimination diet may experience uncomfortable symptoms caused by detoxification, including headache, muscle pains, or fatigue. These symptoms typically appear two to three days into the diet, and disappear within seven days.

When following an elimination diet, be aware that many processed foods contain at least one of the most common food allergens. Milk, soy, wheat, peanuts, and eggs are staples in the food industry, and often appear in foods as "natural flavors," which means that the food label may not list the ingredient.

When it comes to highly processed foods, or sauces and condiments, you will find that allergy avoidance becomes more difficult, because gluten is not always so easy to spot. Soy sauce, for example, often contains gluten as a key ingredient as does teriyaki sauce and food starch.

Gluten-Containing Products[65]

WHEN AVOIDING GLUTEN IN AN ELIMINATION DIET OR ONCE A GLUTEN SENSITIVITY IS DISCOVERED, THE PRODUCTS ON THIS LIST SHOULD BE AVOIDED.

THE FOLLOWING GRAINS AND STARCHES CONTAIN GLUTEN:	THE FOLLOWING INGREDIENTS ARE OFTEN CODE FOR GLUTEN:
Wheat	Avena sativa Cyclodextrin
Wheat germ	Dextrin
Rye	Fermented grain extract
Barley	Hordeum distichon
Bulgur	Hordeum vulgare
Couscous	Hydrolysate
Farina	Hydrolyzed malt extract
Graham flour	Hydrolyzed vegetable protein
Kamut Matzo	Maltodextrin
Semolina	Phytosphingosine extract
Spelt	Samino peptide complex
Triticale	Secale cereale
THE FOLLOWING ARE MISCELLANEOUS SOURCES OF GLUTEN:	Triticum aestivum
shampoos	Triticum vulgare
cosmetics	Tocopherol/vitamin E
lipsticks, lip balm	Yeast extract
Play-Doh	Natural flavoring
medications	Brown rice syrup
non self-adhesive stamps and envelopes	Modified food starch
vitamins and supplements (check label)	Hydrolyzed vegetable protein (HVP)
	Hydrolyzed soy protein
	Caramel color (frequently made from barley)

THE FOLLOWING FOODS OFTEN CONTAIN GLUTEN:

malt/malt flavoring	fruit fillings and puddings
commercial soup, bullion and broths	hot dogs
cold cuts	ice cream
French fries (often dusted with flour before freezing)	root beer
processed cheese (e.g., Velveeta)	energy bars
mayonnaise & ketchup	trail mix
malt vinegar	syrups
soy sauce and teriyaki sauces	seitan
salad dressings	wheatgrass
imitation crab meat, bacon, etc	instant hot drinks
egg substitute	flavored coffees and teas
tabbouleh	vodka
sausage	wine coolers
non-dairy creamer	meatballs, meatloaf communion wafers
fried vegetables/tempura	veggie burgers
gravy	roasted nuts
marinades	beer
canned baked beans	oats (unless certified GF)
cereals	oat bran (unless certified GF)
commercially prepared chocolate milk	blue cheeses
breaded foods	

Source: David Perlmutter, M.D.

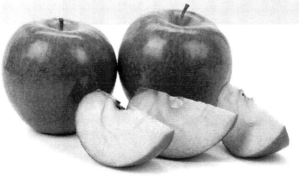

Four steps to gut healing

The four steps to healing leaky gut:

- Remove (irritants)
- Repair (mucosal barrier)
- Replenish (digestive power)
- Restore (bacteria)

Removing irritants from your diet and your environment (work, home, etc.) is critical to setting yourself up for success. Imagine trying to heal from poison ivy while continuing to rub the plant on your skin.

While this step is critical, it can also feel daunting. Don't let that keep you from taking the first step. The elimination diet is your key tool in discovering what foods need to be removed from your diet in order to give yourself the time to heal. This step entails removing all the commercial processed food from your diet.

Complete the ten-day elimination diet and journal your experience. Keep any offending foods out of your diet for three months or longer. You can re-challenge any offending foods once you've completed the gut healing protocol. Ideally, you will continue eating a diet rich in whole-foods. Most people will feel so well after completed the elimination diet that they choose not to reintroduce certain foods. If an "accidental re-introduction" happens during a social event or restaurant meal you will know it. If so, remain committed until the inflammation resolves which can last several days to several weeks.

During this step you will also scan your life for any potential chemicals that are inhibiting your ability to feel your best. Refer back to Part II to review the main environmental triggers and how they may be affecting you and begin transitioning to a safer environment.

Replenishing your digestive power is getting the most of every meal. You want to reduce the stress on your digestive system while your body is healing. Digestive enzymes can be an extremely powerful tool in helping you reduce food sensitivities, absorb nutrients from your foods, and improve overall digestion and elimination.

Replenishing adequate stomach acid is also key, as this ensures proper breakdown of food in the stomach and takes the burden off the small intestines. Consider the use of bitters or supplementing with HCL, especially when you eat animal protein, as discussed in the digestive section.

This step can begin at the same time or soon after step one. In fact, doing so will accelerate your healing process. Most people will continue with step two for up to two months. Digestive symptoms of gas, bloating, flatulence, heartburn, poor elimination or other symptoms would warrant additional time in the replenish stage.

Repairing the mucosal barrier can be accomplished with food and specific supplements. Key gut-healing nutrients and foods include:

- Bone Broth
- Coconut
- L-Glutamine
- Licorice Root (DGL)
- Omega-3 (Fish Oil)

- Zinc
- Curcumin
- Boswellia
- Aloe Vera

Bone broth contains both collagen and amino acids that can help heal your damaged mucosal barrier (gut wall). Coconut products are good for the gut, including coconut oil, which has medium-chain fatty acids (MCFAs) that are easier to digest than other fats and better for leaky gut. Coconut oil is also antifungal and antibacterial, which can help repair and clean up infections.

The amino acid L-Glutamine is one of the most beneficial and widely used supplements for gut repair. It's promotes the repair and growth of your intestinal lining. The recommended dosage is 2–5 grams per day. I suggest the powder form.

Licorice Root (DGL) is an herb that can support the health of the mucosal barrier by helping to balance cortisol levels if you are prone to emotional stress. It has also been shown to improve acid production in the stomach.

One of the main causes of leaky gut is inflammation. Omega-3 fatty acids are comprised of EPA and DHA found in fish and fish oil and are known to combat inflammation. These essential fats are not made by the body and must be eaten or taken in supplement form to ensure the body functions properly. In addition to their anti-inflammatory qualities, these fatty acids support heart health, brain, skins and bone function. You can naturally increase the amount of omega-3 in your diet by eating more fatty fish like salmon, or by taking a high quality fish oil supplement (to avoid mercury and other toxins). When it comes to fish oils, quality matters.

I discussed the risks of zinc deficiency in Part II of this book but in simplest terms a zinc deficiency can lead to inadequate enzyme function and a susceptibility to infection and inflammation in the gut. Research shows that zinc supplementation has tightened leaky gut in people with Crohn's disease.[66]

Anti-inflammatory herbal formulas can also help reduce inflammation and promote gut healing. Look for herbs like turmeric (curcumin) aloe vera, ginger and boswellia (Frankincense). You can find these herbs in formulas or by themselves as part of your overall healing regime. We used frankincense essential oil as part of our gut healing protocol with great success. As always, consult with a nutrition practitioner to determine the dosages and herbs that would be most beneficial to you.

The length of time needed for complete gut repair will vary person to person. It depends on the extent of damage, the level of commitment, and other lifestyle factors that play a role in recovery like sleep and stress management.

Restore your inner-ecosystem. Your gut bacteria play a vital role in keeping you healthy. Restoring the good bacteria in the gut will help you heal and keep you strong going forward.

Probiotics are live bacteria that improve the intestinal microbial balance and enhance overall health. They are the "good" bacteria found in the gastrointestinal track that crowd out the bad bacteria. Inflammation or toxins in the gut can disrupt the natural balance. High-quality probiotics can also assist in the removal of toxins created by gluten sensitivity or celiac disease. In addition, a preventative dose of probiotics is an ideal way to support the immune system going forward.

High quality probiotics can be found in fermented foods that are naturally probiotic rich or in therapeutic-grade supplements with a daily dose of at least ten billion (or more) live, viable, organisms per gram.

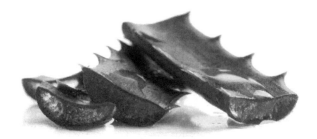

GET AN OIL CHANGE

Choosing the correct oil for cooking or raw consumption can be confusing with all the choices available today. Understanding at what temperature various oils start to smoke and degenerate can help to make decisions easier.

When oil is heated to a high temperature, it reaches its smoke point. The bluish smoke that can then be seen means the oil is close to burning and is the temperature at which fats and oils begin to break down. Nutritional degradation and the chemical composition of the oil changes at this point, sometimes with effects that are harmful to your health. A low smoke point means the oil should not be used for cooking. A high smoke point oil can be used for cooking at higher temperatures, for example pan frying.

OLIVE OIL

The smoke point for olive oil varies considerably and is based on the quality of the oils and the way in which the oil has been extracted. Extra virgin, virgin and extra light oils all have different qualities, but all are high in monounsaturated fat, making them heart healthy. Olive oil has a relatively high smoke point (the more refined it is, the higher the smoke point). Extra virgin olive oil breaks down at a lower temperature and is, therefore, best kept for uncooked uses like salad dressing.

- EXTRA VIRGIN OLIVE OIL: 320 degrees F (160 C)

- VIRGIN OLIVE OIL: 420 degrees F (216 C)

- EXTRA LIGHT: 468 degrees F (242 C)

COCONUT OIL

Coconut oil is extracted from fresh coconuts and tolerates a fairly high temperature, making it safe to use for cooking. Smoke point is 350 degrees F (177°C).

WALNUT OIL

Unrefined walnut oil has a smoke point of 320 degrees F (160°C). It is, therefore, easily damaged when heated to a high temperature. Walnut oil is best used in small amounts, for salads and salad dressings. It has a rich nutty flavor.

Macadamia nut oil has a high heat capacity with a smoke point of 413 degrees F (210°C). It contains up to eighty-five percent monounsaturated fats and has a shelf life of around two years. It's a good choice for stir-fry dishes, searing, or baking.

The following nutrient-rich traditional fats have nourished healthy population groups for thousands of years:[67]

CONFUSED ABOUT WHAT FATS/OILS TO USE?

FOR COOKING:

- Butter
- Tallow from beef or lamb
- Lard from pigs
- Chicken, goose or duck fat
- Coconut, palm and palm kernel oils

FOR SALADS:

- Extra virgin olive oil
- Expeller-expressed sesame and peanut oils
- Expeller-expressed flax oil (in small amounts)

THE FOLLOWING FATS CAN CAUSE CANCER, HEART DISEASE, IMMUNE SYSTEM DYSFUNCTION, STERILITY, LEARNING DISABILITIES, GROWTH PROBLEMS, AND OSTEOPOROSIS:

- All hydrogenated and partially hydrogenated oils
- Industrially processed liquid oils, such as corn, soy, safflower, cottonseed and canola
- Fats and oils (especially vegetable oils) heated to very high temperatures in processing and frying.

Source: Weston A. Price Foundation

Traditional foods and techniques

Modern convenience has led to the abandonment of traditional foods. Most of what is available today, whether from the market or restaurant, is either highly processed or made with ingredients that are themselves highly processed.

Traditional foods take time, but the health benefits make them well worth it. Examples of traditional foods include: sprouted and fermented grains, fermented vegetables, cultured dairy, organ meats, and bone broth. These may all seem foreign to you, but for many they are foods our grandparents made and when we think back to our childhood, we may remember their place in the home. Here are some of my favorite traditional foods and techniques and the benefits to including them in your diet.

Bone Broth

- It is full of minerals

- It enhances digestion by healing the gut lining.

- It nourishes all parts of the body related to collagen. This means joints, tendons, ligaments, skin, mucus membranes, and bone.

Bones are highly mineralized. A homemade bone broth will deliver your body calcium, phosphorous, magnesium, sodium, potassium, sulfate, and fluoride—in a form that your body understands.

Bones, marrow, skin, tendons, ligaments, and the cartilage that sometimes accompanies a bone are all made of a protein molecule called collagen. Collagen contains two very special amino acids: proline and glycine.

Collagen has been found to help heal the lining of the gastrointestinal tract, which includes the stomach and the intestines. This means that if you suffer from symptoms of intestinal inflammation like heartburn or GERD (gastroesophageal reflux disease) bone broth can help. In addition to collagen, cartilage also contains gelatin which has been shown to benefit gastric ulcers.[68]

Besides collagen, cartilage contains something called glycosaminoglycans (GAGs). Studies have found an underlying deficiency of glycosaminoglycans (GAGs) in patients with Crohn's and ulcerative colitis. Correcting a deficiency and helping to repair a compromised gut wall is another good reason to consume bone broth regularly.[69]

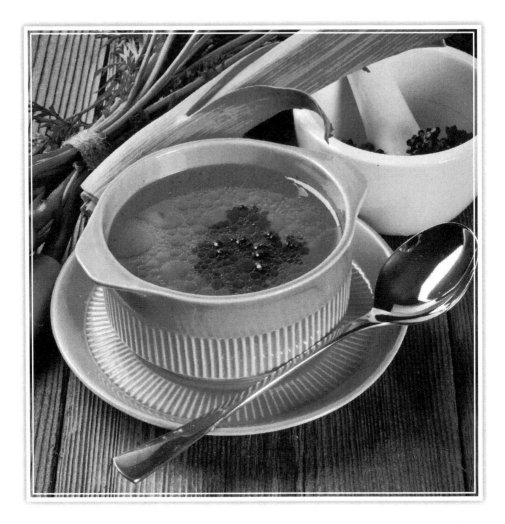

Wrinkles, stretch marks, and cellulite, oh my! The smoothness of your skin comes from connective tissue. Bone broth makes skin supple. Cellulite is not from excess fat. We all know thin people with cellulite. Cellulite comes from a lack of connective tissue. Collagen-rich bone broth will supply your skin with the tools it need to support itself.

How to make it

Go for variety when collecting bone, but any kind will do. The marrow found in bones is either yellow marrow or red marrow. Yellow marrow is found in the central portion of long bones. It is where fats are stored. Red marrow, on the other hand, is found in flat bones. These are: hip bone, sternum, skull, ribs, vertebrae, scapula, and the ends of long bones.

Red marrow is so valuable because it is where blood stem cells are found. When you drink a broth made with a good source of red marrow, you are drinking all those stem cell factors that ultimately build your body's strength and support your own immune function.

Quality matters. Make sure that all bones are sourced from animals that are organic and grass-fed or pastured and free-range. Remember, everything that the animal ate, how it lived, and where it lived all factor into the health benefits of your broth. You would not want to consume broth made from the bones of an animal that was factory-farmed, treated with steroids and antibiotics, confined, and fed GMO corn or soy. Animals that are pastured, eating grass and exposed to natural sunlight are healthy.

You can purchase bones ready to cook from your local famer or at a natural food market, or you can collect bones from meals and store them in your freezer until you have enough to build a good stock. If you are using large bones, ask the butcher to cut them into smaller pieces. This reduces cooking time and allows more material to become a part of the broth.

Cooking Suggestions

1. Place chicken or beef bones into a large stock pot and cover with water. Fill the pot with filtered water and leave plenty of room for water to boil.

2. Add two tablespoon of apple cider vinegar or wine to water prior to cooking. The acidity helps pull out important nutrients from the bones.

3. Bring to a boil and remove any scum as it rises, then reduce heat to simmer for a minimum of six hours. Chicken bones can cook for six to forty-eight hours. I usally cook mine for thirty-six hours. Beef bones can cook for twelve to seventy-two hours. A long and slow cook time is necessary in order to fully extract the nutrients in and around bone. If you don't have a gas stove, use a crock pot. You will not be able to control temperature with an electric stovetop.

After cooking, allow the broth to cool and transfer to several glass mason jars. Leave about an inch of room at the top for expansion if you plan to store in the freezer (I learned that the hard way!) A layer of fat will harden on top once it's refrigerated. This layer protects the broth beneath. Discard this layer only when you are about to eat the broth. Consume broth within one to two weeks or freeze for later use. We use our broth to make risotto, homemade soups or to cook rice (in place of using plain water). If anyone is sick we make a healing elixer with warm broth, ginger, lemon and parsley.

Soaking & Sprouting

Nuts, grains, seeds, and legumes

Our ancestor understood instinctively that nuts are best soaked and/or sprouted before you eat them. Nuts contain numerous enzyme inhibitors that can strain the digestive system.

Nutritional inhibitors and toxic substances found in nuts, grains and seed are nature's defense but can be minimized or eliminated by soaking. These inhibitors and toxic substances are known as **enzyme inhibitors** and **phytates** (phytic acid).

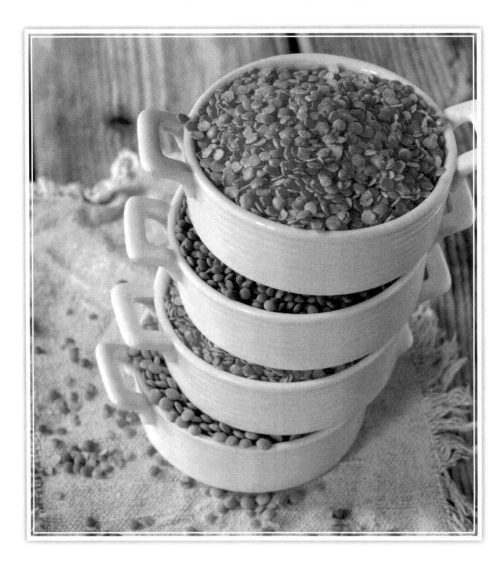

Nature has set it up so that nuts, grains and seeds may survive until proper growing conditions are present. When it rains they gets wet and can then germinate to produce a plant. So we are mimicking nature when we soak our nuts, grains and seeds.

What are Enzyme inhibitors?

There are digestive enzymes and metabolic enzymes. Digestive enzymes help break down food. Metabolic enzymes help every biological process the body performs. Enzyme inhibitors will clog, warp, or denature an active site of an enzyme. They may also bind to the enzyme, which will prevent the intended molecule from binding. This leads to poor digestion.

What are Phytates?

All grains contain phytic acid in the outer layer or bran. Untreated phytic acid can combine with calcium, magnesium, copper, iron and especially zinc in the intestinal tract and block their absorption. This is known as chelation and can be very problematic for people with existing mineral deficiencies, like children on the autism spectrum.

This is why diets high in unfermented whole grains may lead to serious mineral deficiencies and bone loss. The modern practice of consuming large amounts of processed foods and improperly prepared grains could have long-term health effects on many people.

Soaking and Sprouting

I soak my nuts, grains, and seeds in filtered water with a tablespoon of something acidic like apple cider vinegar or lemon juice. In some cases, I use just filtered water. Within seven to twenty-four hours most enzyme inhibitors are neutralized and the anti-nutrients are broken down.

If you choose to consume nuts, grains and seeds wet, make smaller batches and store them in the refrigerator. Usually everything that is soaked is dried in a dehydrator or oven on the lowest possible setting for twenty-four to forty-eight hours to remove all moisture. Otherwise you will develop mold.

You can also dry sprouted nuts, seeds and grains in a low-temperature oven or dehydrator, and then grind them in your grain mill or food processor and use as a flour in a variety of recipes.

Soaking and Sprouting Chart

Product	Dry Amount	Soaking Time	Sprouting Time	Yield	Additional Comments
Alfalfa seeds	3 tbls	5 hours	4–5 days	4 cups	Place sprouts in direct sunlight on the last day of sprouting to "green" them and increase their chlorophyll content.
Almonds	3 cups	24–48 hours	–	4 cups	Almonds just need to be soaked for 1–2 days and then kept in the refrigerator in water. Change water daily. Will keep for 5–6 days.
All other nuts—walnuts, macadamia, etc.	3 cups	6–8 hours	–	4 cups	These nuts will not sprout. They just need to be soaked and then used or kept in the refrigerator for a day or two.
Amaranth	1 cup	3–4 hours	1–2 days	3 cups	Rinse 3–4 times per day. These small seeds sprout very quickly.
Barley (hulled)*	1 cup	6 hours	12–24 hours	2 cups	Rinse 3–4 times a day.
Buckwheat (hulled)	1 cup	6 hours	1–2 days	2 cups	Rinse 3–4 times a day.
Clover	3 tbls	5 hours	5 days	4 cups	Place sprouts in direct sunlight on the last day of sprouting to "green" them and increase their chlorophyll content.
Fenugreek Seeds	4 tbls	6 hours	4–5 days	3 cups	The longer the sprout the more bitter it becomes.
Flax seeds	1 cup	6 hours	–	2 cups	Flax seeds will soak up a large amount of water so make sure you give them enough to absorb. They do not need to be sprouted, just soaked.
Lentil	¾ cup	8 hours	3 days	4 cups	Rinse 2–3 times a day.
Garbanzo Bean (chick peas)	1 cup	12 hours	3 days	4 cups	Rinse 3–4 times a day.

Product	Dry Amount	Soaking Time	Sprouting Time	Yield	Additional Comments
Millet	1 cup	5 hours	12 hours	3 cups	These small seeds sprout very quickly. The sprout will be very small on these.
Mung Beans	⅓ cup	8 hours	4–5 days	4 cups	Rinse these sprouts vigorously to remove the hulls after sprouted.
Pea	1 cup	8 hours	3 days	3 cups	
Pumpkin seeds	1 cup	6 hours	1 day	2 cups	You don't have to wait for these to sprout. You can use them after soaking.
Quinoa	1 cup	3 hours	1–2 days	3 cups	
Radish	3 tbls	6 hours	4–5 days	4 cups	Place sprouts in direct sunlight on the last day of sprouting to "green" them and increase their chlorophyll content.
Rye berries*	1 cup	6 hours	2–3 days	3 cups	Rinse 2–3 times a day.
Sesame seeds	1 cup	4 hours	1 day	1 cup	Only hulled sesame sees will sprout.
Spelt*	1 cup	6 hours	1–2 days	3 cups	Can be used as a substitute for wheat.
Sunflower seeds	1 cup	6 hours	1 day	2 cups	You don't have to wait for these to sprout. You can use them after soaking.
Teff	1 cup	3 hours	1–2 days	3 cups	
Wheat berries* **Note:** use the soft wheat berries for bread and crackers and hard wheat berries for wheat grass.	1 cup	8 hours	2–3 days	3 cups	Rinse 3–4 times a day.
Wild rice	1 cup	12 hours	2–3 days	3 cups	Make sure you use <u>wild</u> rice.

* Contains gluten. Avoid if eating a gluten-free diet.

Source: Living on Live Food by Alissa Cohen

Nut Milks

Once you become accustomed to soaking nuts, you can also experiment with making your own nut milks. There are several varieties of nut milk on the market now, most of which are highly processed and full of sugar. The most common are almond, cashew and hazelnut. Almond milk in particular is high in protein and magnesium, which is good for bone strength.

Nut milks are so simple to make. Almond milk is a great base for homemade granola, smoothies, and milkshakes, or added to tea or coffee. Here's what you'll need:

- 1 cup raw almonds

- 4 cups filtered water

- Small pinch of sea salt

- A dash of organic vanilla extract

- 1 tsp of maple syrup or raw honey if you want it sweet (optional)

- Blender

1. Soak the nuts for eight hours in filtered water and rinse thoroughly. You can "peel" the almonds if you want white, pure milk with absolutely no enzyme-inhibitors. If so, simply pinch the soaked almonds in between your fingertips and the shell will slip off.

2. Add the four cups of filtered water into high-speed blender and all other ingredients. Blend until smooth. That's it!

Optional: If you want a thin milk, strain the pulp through a nut milk bag into a bowl, squeezing out the liquid through with your hands or through a fine mesh cloth. I like it a little thicker so I don't strain. I do have to add a little extra water though. Keeps well in refrigerator for three to four days. Store in an airtight mason jar.

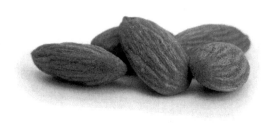

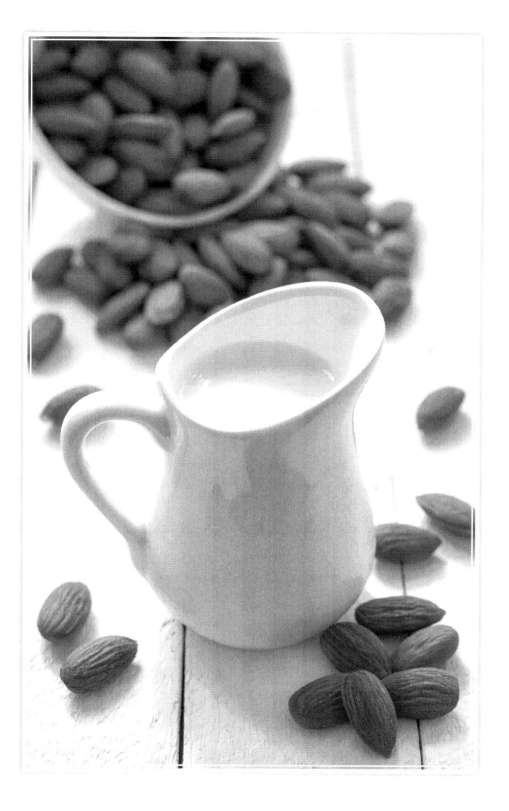

Fermented Foods—Nature's Probiotics

Kimchi (or kimchee), sauerkraut, and kombucha are some of the world's great fermented foods. A fermented food is one whose taste and texture have been transformed by the introduction of beneficial bacteria or fungi. They were a part of traditional diets.

Before I switched to a real food diet, foods like sauerkraut, kimchi and kombucha were foreign to me. These foods taste and smell strong but pack healing power.

Fermented foods are foods that have been through a process of lacto-fermentation in which natural bacteria feed on the sugar and starch in the food creating lactic acid. This process preserves the food, and creates beneficial enzymes, B vitamins and various strains of probiotics (bacteria).

Natural fermentation of foods has also been shown to preserve nutrients in food and break the food down to a more digestible form. This could explain the link between a diet rich in fermented foods and improved digestion.

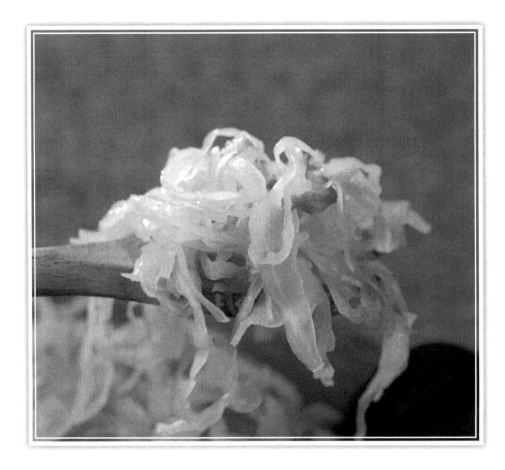

Cultures around the world have been eating fermented foods for years. Studies show a link between probiotic-rich foods and overall health. Sadly, with the advances in technology and food preparation, these time-honored traditional foods have been largely lost in our society.

The amount of probiotics and enzymes available in the average diet has declined drastically over the last few decades as pasteurized milk has replaced raw, pasteurized yogurt has replaced homemade, and vinegar based pickles and sauerkraut have replaced traditional lacto-fermented versions.

BENEFITS TO FERMENTED FOODS

Eating fermented foods and drinking fermented drinks (like kefir and kombucha) will introduce probiotics, also known as beneficial bacteria, into your digestive system and help the balance of good bacteria in your digestive system. Fermented foods are nature's version of probiotics which been shown to improve our health through the following functions:

- Improve bowel movements by regulating peristalsis (contraction of the colon)

- Break down sugar, lactose and oxalates in the diet;

- Balance our intestinal pH

- Makes many of the B vitamins available to the body

- Supports our immune system

For those who are intimidated with the process of fermentation, there are many good products on the market today to experiment with. To learn more about fermenting, consider *Wild Fermentation: The Flavor, Nutrition, and Craft of Live-Culture Foods*, by Sandor Ellix Katz.

And if the idea of eating these pungent foods makes you squirm, consider a therapeutic grade probiotic supplement to deliver the important benefits of bacteria to the gut. There are literally hundreds of strains of bacteria in our body.

Probiotics are essential for life. For those with chronic health issues including autoimmune, it can be one of the most important steps in rebuilding your health. If you are sensitive to casein, be sure to choose a strain that does not contain milk. There are also strains such as saccharomyces boulardii (or S. boulardii), which are yeast that kills candida. This strain can be found in some formulations. I use Ortho Molecular Ortho Biotic which has the S. boulardii strain.

Kombucha is a cultured beverage that is our version of "soda." It is a brew of sweetened tea (black or green) that is fermented with a culture of bacteria and yeast. The bacteria and yeast feed off the sugar turning this simple tea into a healing elixir capable of combating constipations, candida overgrowth, digestive issues, detoxification and immune function.

The beneficial strains of yeast and bacteria in kombucha, lactobacillus and saccharomyces, also inhibit pathogenic microbes such staphylococcus, e. coli, salmonella, listeria and helicobacter pylori (H. Pylori). In this case, the beneficial yeast kill yeast in the body, rather than feed it as you would experience with sugar.

You may be sensitive to kombucha if you react to phenols, which are high in tea. One way to combat that sensitivity and reap the benefits of the kombucha would be to take a digestive enzyme that specifically targets at breaking down phenols. I use No Fenol by Houston Enzymes.

Like any health food, the Internet is full of lists with promising benefits of anything from weight loss to radiant skin. Fortunately, kombucha has been around a long time and has much to show in terms of its healing qualities:

- Inhibits harmful bacteria

- Repairs tissue and provides amino acids, the building blocks to your cells

- Helps digestion and relieves constipation

- Fights infections such as candida and thrush

- Detoxification—happy liver equals happy mood

- Cell regeneration

- Supports cellular energy production

You can find kombucha at most health food stores (although it is expensive). This year I will be making my own at home. If you are interested in making it yourself, you can buy a complete kit online at www.kombuchakamp.com.

OIL PULLING

Oil pulling is "all the craze" right now. Seems like every week there is a new post in social media about oil pulling and the magical wonders it provides. It begs the question: Are the benefits of oil pulling myth or fact?

I first learned about oil pulling when I was studying traditional Ayurvedic remedies. It is an ancient practice of swishing oil around the mouth in order to cleanse toxins from the body and the mouth. It's used for common oral mouth issues, like bleeding gums, canker sores, tooth decay, and detoxification.[70]

Here's how it works: You simply take one tablespoon of sesame oil or coconut oil in your mouth the first thing in the morning immediately after waking (before eating). Swish the oil around the mouth for up to twenty minutes and then spit it out. Do not swallow the oil. Rinse the mouth and brush your teeth. The traditional method suggests sesame oil but in cases of bacterial overgrowth or oral mouth issues, coconut oil makes a better choice because of its antibacterial properties.

As I looked to the research on the benefits of oil pulling, many reference to the "extensive use as a traditional Indian folk remedy to prevent teeth decay, oral malodor, bleeding gums, dryness of throat and cracked lips, and for strengthening the teeth, gums, and jaws." New scientific findings were promising, with studies on evaluating the effect of oil pulling with sesame oil on the count of Streptococcus mutans in plaque and saliva of children.[71]

ORAL HEALTH BENEFITS:

- Strengthen mouth and gums
- Prevent gum bleeding, cavities and gingivitis
- Brighter teeth and prevents yellowing
- Remove plague
- Relieves toothaches

BENEFITS BEYOND THE MOUTH:

- Reduces inflammation
- Helps detoxify the body
- Heals skin conditions
- Reduces body pain
- Reduces chest congestion
- Support immunity
- Balances hormones
- Relieves seasonal allergies
- Improves vision

PLANT-BASED MEDICINE CABINET

Essential oils are natural compounds found in the seeds, bark, stems, roots, flowers, and other parts of plants. In addition to giving plants their distinctive smells, essential oils provide plants with protection against predators and disease and play a role in plant pollination.

Essential oils are fat-soluble although they do not include fatty lipids or acids found in vegetable and animal oils. Essential oils are very clean, almost crisp, to the touch and are immediately absorbed by the skin.

> **TRY THIS AT HOME**
>
> Squeeze the peel of a ripe orange. The fragrant residue on your hand is full of essential oils.

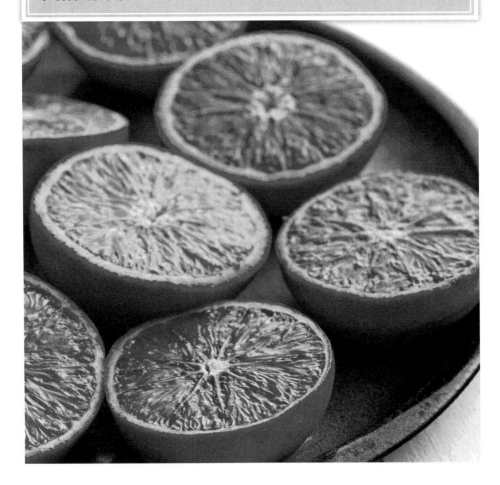

Essential oils are used widely as natural medicine but without the side effects of conventional drugs like aspirin and antibiotics. Having a plant-based first aid kit for wounds, stings, sunburns, aches and pains have served me well with three little boys.

HERE IS WHAT MY FIRST-AID KIT INCLUDES:

- LAVENDER: Burns, cuts, rashes, stings, reduce anxiety, sleep and all things calming.

- PEPPERMINT: Relieves pain in joints, muscles, relieve digestive issues, reduce fevers, clear sinuses, improve asthma, bronchitis and relieve headaches.

- FRANKINCENSE: Anti-inflammatory, heal bruising, reduce scars, boost immunity.

- MELALEUCA (TEA TREE OIL): Anti-bacterial, anti-fungal, skin irritations, itchy rashes.

- CLOVE: Anti-oxidant, healthy teeth and gums.

- EUCALYPTUS: Respiratory health, sore muscles, coughs, sore throat.

THE MOST COMMON ESSENTIAL OILS—LAVENDER, FRANKINCENSE, LEMON, PEPPERMINT, AND TEA TREE OIL—HAVE BEEN USED FOR COMMON AILMENTS LIKE:

- Fight cold and flu symptoms

- Relaxation, insomnia, or stress relief

- Skin conditions—acne, eczema or bug bites

- Pain relief from exercise or injuries

- Digestive symptom relief and stomach aches

- Disinfectants and safe cleaning products

- Anti-fungal and anti-bacterial treatment

The therapeutic benefits are delivered to our cells due to the small molecular size of the oils which are able to penetrate into the cells in our body and some believe that certain compounds can even cross the blood-brain barrier.

Most people are familiar with the use of essential oils in lotions, candles and other personal care products. Today, many professionals, like massage therapist, physical therapists, nutritionists, naturopathic doctors, and even hospitals, use essential oils as non-invasive way to ease symptoms of illness during treatment.

The Vanderbilt University Medical Center in Nashville, Tennessee, uses them in the treatment of anxiety, depression and infections. A 2009 study found that pre-operative patients who received aromatherapy with lavender oil were significantly less anxious about their surgery than controls.[72] Other oils have been used successfully to decrease symptoms of nausea.[73] A 2007 study in the *Journal of Alternative and Complementary Medicine* suggests that women who used aromatherapy during labor reported less pain overall and were able to use fewer pain medications.

EACH AND EVERY ESSENTIAL OIL CONTAINS COMPOUNDS WITH UNIQUE HEALING AND THERAPEUTIC BENEFITS. HERE ARE MY TOP FIVE OILS BEYOND THE FIRST-AID KIT AND HOW TO USE THEM.

- GINGER: Reduces inflammation, supports joints, improves digestion and relieves nausea.[74] We make a great ginger ale at home with sparkling mineral water, ginger oil, lemon and raw honey.

- LEMON: Cleanses the body by improving lymphatic drainage and antioxidant.[75] Also great to use in homemade cleaning products.

- MYRRH: Natural anti-septic and can prevent or reduce infections.[76] It's been show to support beautiful skin, reduces stretch marks and promotes hormone balance. Also used as anti-inflammatory.[77]

- OREGANO: Powerful anti-microbial properties.[78] Also shown to kill fungus and parasites.[79]

- ROSEMARY: Therapeutic benefits in prevention of asthma, peptic ulcer, inflammatory diseases and more.[80]

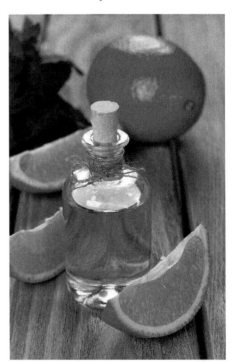

HERE ARE THE FOUR MOST COMMON WAYS THAT ESSENTIAL OILS CAN USE USED FOR OVERALL WELLNESS:

- TOPICALLY: Apply to the bottom of feet. According to scientific testing, essential oils can pass through the skins and into the blood stream making them very effective and easy to apply.

- AROMATICALLY: Breathe! There is great evidence that essential oils are absorbed when inhaled due to the large volume of blood vessels in the lungs to absorb them. A diffuser can also help you experience the benefits of essential oils

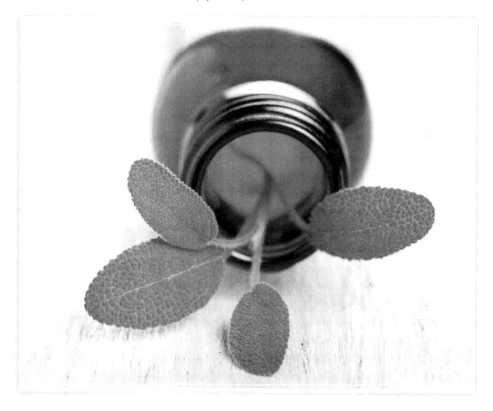

- INGESTION: Not all essential oils are created equal. Be sure to only ingest those oils that are safe for internal use and are clearly labeled for this use. Essential oils are powerful and a little goes a long way (less than five drops mixed with water is very effective).

Oils like peppermint, lemon, and frankincense have great internal benefits and can be taken with water. Other essential oils like clove and oregano need to be diluted and should only taken internally for a short period (less than ten days).

- **PERSONAL CARE:** After reading about environmental triggers, I imagine you are feeling frustrated with all the toxins on the market today. Once I became informed of the potential dangers, I felt motivated to jump onto the do-it-yourself bandwagon. Today, the fastest way essential oils are being used is by making homemade personal care products. This is an excellent way to take advantage of essential oils to improve your beauty, home and long-term health. Some of my favorite DIY products to make at home include bug repellant, deodorant, and household cleaning products.

  For oils that require dilution or "carrier" oil, I recommend coconut or olive oil.

- **CONTRAINDICATIONS:** Because essential oils can act as a powerful form of natural medicine, there are a few instances where they are not recommended for usage: Pregnancy: Avoid basil, cinnamon, clary sage, clove, cypress, fennel, jasmine, juniper, marjoram, myrrh, rose, rosemary, sage and thyme. Heart medications (blood thinners): Avoid clary sage, cypress, eucalyptus, ginger, rosemary, sage and thyme. Always consult your healthcare practitioner before use.

- **QUALITY:** Not all essential oils are created equally. In fact, there are many brands that are synthetic and therefore provide no health benefits. When purchasing essential oils, always make sure they are certified pure therapeutic grade.

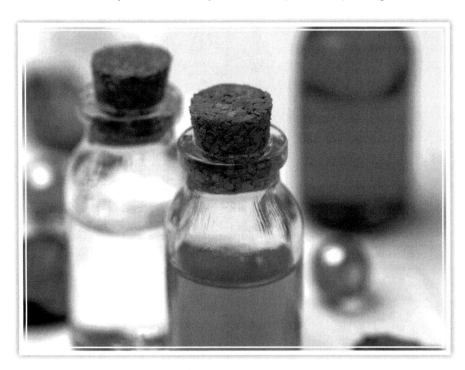

Part III: Action Takeaways

A ten-day elimination diet is one of the most effective ways
to determine if you have food sensitivities.
It will change your life!

. . . .

There are four steps to healing the gut and rebuilding your
foundation of health (your immune system): (1) Remove irritants,
(2) Replenish your digestive power, (3) Repair the mucosal barrier,
and (4) Restore your inner ecosystem with beneficial bacteria.

. . . .

Traditional foods and techniques have a long history of nourishing
our bodies and building strong immune systems.

. . . .

Nutritional inhibitors can be found on healthy foods.
Learn the techniques that our ancestors used
to get the most nutrition from our foods.

. . . .

Add fermented foods to your diet—
Mother Nature's version of probiotics.

. . . .

Convert your medicine cabinet to a plant-based version
using the healing properties of essential oils.

. . . .

Ask yourself today:

Could an elimination diet help me discover
the missing link to my ongoing health complaints?
(Let me help you with this one. YES!)

. . . .

Am I properly preparing nuts, seeds and grains?

. . . .

Am I using over-the-counter or prescription medications
for aches and pains without considering the healing properties
and safety of essential oils first?

. . . .

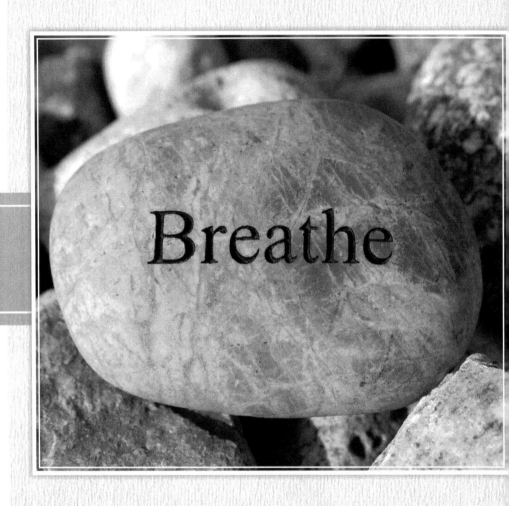

PART IV: PREVENTION

Creating the "Toolbox" for Self-care

> *If you think you can, or you think you can't, you're right*
> ~ Henry Ford

You must take personal responsibility for your own life and your choices. Once you have become your own nutrition detective and eliminated the foods and other triggers keeping you from feeling your best, it will be the consistency of your choices that presents the initial challenge.

Inevitably you will be challenged. It will happen at holidays, social events, restaurants, and cookouts—essentially anywhere people gather around food. You will be questioned, berated, criticized and even teased about what you are "not" eating. And you can, and should, hold your ground.

Here are the three phases that you can anticipate from others in response to your new-found health: Ridicule, resistance, and acceptance. People like to make fun of things they don't fully understand. For example people love to claim "the gluten free diet is a fad." Fortunately, there is a growing body of research and extensive amount of personal stories and experience that confirm the devastating impact of gluten on our health. It's always best to stay informed, know the facts and consider that many people gather their data and form opinions based on the latest media headline or outdated information rather than the actual research.

After ridicule, comes resistance. This is where you get the push back. My husband and children skipped stage one and moved right into stage two where they stayed the longest. Our initial introduction to gluten-free living was presented as a thirty-day challenge. I made the announcement and everyone hemmed and hawed but ultimately agreed. After all, it was ONLY thirty days, or so they thought.

Soon the thirty days passed and everyone was still alive. Shocking, I know. I continued to maintain a gluten-free kitchen. Then the birthday parties and special occasions rolled around and the menu planning began. Who will be bringing what? Of course I announced we would be setting boundaries around what others could bring and that's when my husband blurted out, "How long do we plan to live like this?" There it was—the tip of the resistance iceberg. Although I felt irritated inside, I calmly replied, "What exactly are you missing that you can't live without?" He paused and said, "Nothing, I guess". The truth is, we were still eating all our favorite foods, including some of the "comfort" foods and desserts—lasagna, pancakes, and brownies—but I was making them without the gluten.

Then we had the "safe haven" talk. My youngest son has a life-threatening immune response to peanuts, and glycoproteins found in the saliva of dogs and cats. He would have an allergic reaction that would result in anaphylaxis if he ate peanuts. We would have to administer epinephrine to save his life. Needless to say, we don't allow peanuts (or dogs or cats) in our home. This is simple for anyone to understand.

In the case of my oldest son and myself, our immune response to gluten is delayed. We would not require epinephrine however we would trigger an autoimmune response in the body that would have a dramatic effect on our health. In fact, a recent study in the *Journal of the American Medical Association* of 30,000 patients found that people diagnosed with full blown celiac, undiagnosed celiac (inflammation to their intestines), and those with "latent" celiac disease or gluten sensitivity (elevated gluten antibodies but negative intestinal biopsy) had a higher risk of death, from heart disease and cancer.[81] The findings were dramatic. There was a thirty-nine percent increased risk of death in those with celiac disease, seventy-two percent increased risk in those with gut inflammation related to gluten, and thirty-five percent increased risk in those with gluten sensitivity but no celiac disease.

This is ground-breaking research that proves you don't have to have full-blown celiac disease with a positive intestinal biopsy (which is what conventional thinking tells us) to have serious health problems and complications—even death—from eating gluten. This led me to my next questions: Why should I put any member of my family at risk in our own home? That was the birth of our safe haven. I made a pact with myself that I would not compromise the health of ANY family member over any food ingredient on the market. Ever.

What I learned from this experience was that the whole family developed a much broader interest in food. We began inventing recipes in an attempt to re-create some of our favorite foods. We made granola cereal and bars from an assortment of nuts and seeds (peanuts are legumes, not nuts). We made chocolate chips cookies, home-made ice-cream, lasagna with zucchini noodles, meatballs, veggies roll-ups, and our family favorite—chocolate protein balls from hemp, cashew butter and cacao. We were eating real food. We had graduated (albeit reluctantly) to the acceptance stage.

Convincing others, like relatives and friends, will take patience and strength. It can be tempting to give into the "what's the big deal?" or "one bite won't kill you" comments. But if you have an autoimmune disease, food sensitivity, or if you just want to avoid foods that make you feel lousy, then saying no is in your power. Don't compromise your boundaries to please others because the person you will let down in the process is yourself. It's nobody's job to take care of you, except you.

PLANNING IS KEY

TO HANDLE SOCIAL SITUATIONS WITH GRACE CONSIDER THIS:

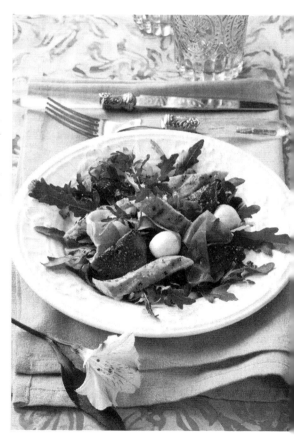

When you are invited to share a meal or a special occasion outside your home, call family or friends in advance and tell them of your dietary restrictions. Recognize that they may feel overwhelmed with the job of finding something to cook for you. This is a chance to brainstorm ideas or to bring along a dish that is safe for you and that others can enjoy too.

A tip to reduce your urge to give in to temptation is to eat before you arrive. The rule in our home is to never leave the house hungry. Even a light healthy snack can give you the strength to stay the course.

CREATING A SAFE HAVEN

TRANSITIONING TO AN "ALLERGEN-FREE" KITCHEN

We maintain a gluten-free, GMO-free, soy-free, peanut-free, chemical-free, and commerically-processed dairy-free kitchen. (Say that five time fast.) You can adjust your kitchen to meet your own dietary requirments. Once you have discarded all the wheat and white flour, cookies, crackers, cereals, commericial dairy products and refined sugars, here are just **some** of the essentials that you want to replace them with.

Please keep in mind that your first few shopping trips will be more expensive as you develop a stable stocked pantry. There may be many foods you simply do not have yet, but as you build inventory, weekly shopping will become more affordable and less overwhelming.

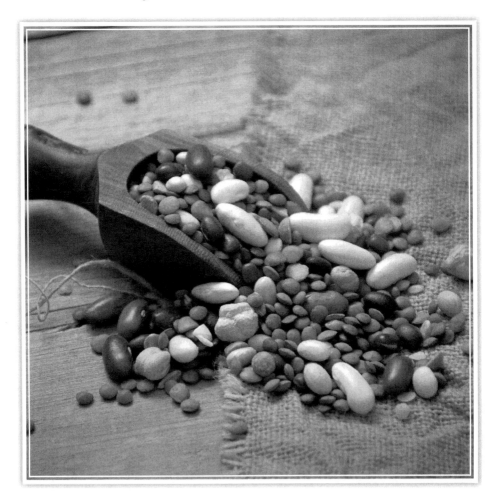

This is a sneak peek at what my pantry includes.

GF GRAINS & STARCHES	VEGGIES	DAIRY & OTHER	BAKING/COOKING	SEASONINGS
Quinoa*	Think Seasonal! Dark Leafy Greens	Coconut Milk	Almond Flour	Apple Cider Vinegar
Brown Rice	Celery	Almond Milk	Coconut Flour	Sea Salt
Buckwheat	Garlic	Organic, cage-free eggs	Baking Soda (aluminum-free)	Coconut Aminos (soy sauce alternative)
GF Bread**	Onions/leeks	Raw, hard cheese	GF Vanilla	Dulse Flakes
Rice Pasta (Jovial)**	Carrots		GF Chicken Broth	Cinnamon
Potatoes	Mushrooms		GF Veggie Broth	Turmeric
Sweet Potatoes	Cucumbers		Pitted Dates	Raw Honey
Organic (or non-GMO)	Broccoli		Raw local honey	Stevia Extract
Tachos	Carrots		Real Maple Syrup	GF Ketchup
Arborio Rice (Risotto)	Brussels sprouts		Choc Chips (Enjoy Life)	GF Mustard
	Squash			Sauerkraut (Bubbies)

* Technically a seed, not a grain
** Transition Foods. Ideally you want to move to a whole food diet, not a GF processed food diet.

SNACKS	NUTS & SEEDS	FRUITS	OILS AND FATS	LEGUMES
GF Crackers**	Cashews	Think Seasonal! Berries	Coconut Oil	Cannellini Beans
GF Tortilla Chips **	Pine Nuts	Apples	EV Olive Oil	Azuki Beans
Hummus	Pistachio	Pears	Avocados	Navy Beans
GF Dark Chocolate	Walnuts	Olives	Kerrygold Butter	Black Beans
Nut Butters	Almonds	Bananas	Proteins	Lentils
Nut Thin crackers	Macadamia	Melon	Grass fed meat	Chick peas
	Pumpkin		Wild caught fish	
	Sunflower		Pasture-raised	
	Chia Seeds		Chicken	
	Flax Seeds		Wild Game	

Note: Eden Organics is currently the only brand that uses BPA-free lining in their cans. Ideally, you want to purchase beans dry, then soak and sprout.

Self-care practices

Sleep

Sleep your way to better health. Now that you have a better understanding of hormones you can better appreciate the impact the sleep has on hormone health and even cancer prevention. Researchers believe this link is caused by differing levels of melatonin in people who are exposed to light at night, like people who work the late shift, and higher rate for breast and colon cancer. Melatonin, the hormone that makes us tired at night and appears to suppress growth of tumors, is reduced with light exposure at night.

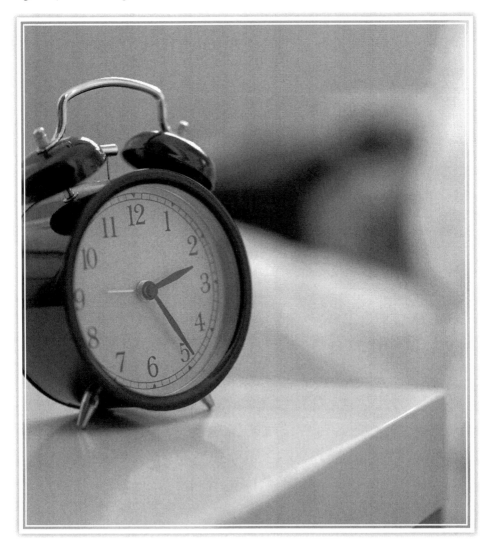

When your body is sleep deprived, it functions in stress mode, which leads to an increase in blood pressure and a production of stress hormones, like cortisol. Higher blood pressure increases your risk for heart attacks and strokes. An increase in cortisol not only makes it harder for you to sleep but also leads to inflammation. Increased inflammation leads to degeneration, injury and early signs of aging.

Research also tells us that people who sleep less than seven hours per night are more likely to be overweight or obese. This lack of sleep impacts the balance of hormones in the body from elevated cortisol to poor regulation of appetite. The production of ghrelin and leptin, hormones that regulate appetite, are disrupted by lack of sleep. So if you are gaining weight or can't lose weight despite good nutrition and movement, consider your sleep patterns before you run for the next dietary theory or weight loss supplement.

SOME PRACTICES THAT WILL ENSURE A GOOD NIGHT'S SLEEP:

- Darken your room to increase melatonin production.

- Remove all technology from the bedroom to reduce Electromagnetic field (EMF) exposure.

- Stop using computers and television at least one hour before bedtime to reduce stimulation.

- Create a bedtime "routine" that promotes relaxation.

- Take a detox bath with Epsom salt (see details below), which provides your body with magnesium sulfate to help relax your muscles and detoxify toxins from the body.

- Read a book, mediate, keep a gratitude journal.

- Apply a few drops of lavender oil to the bottom on your feet or include in your bedtime bath to reduce cortisol, which will lower inflammation and promote weight loss.

- For persistent sleep issues consider the use of amino acids therapy. Many people have disrupted melatonin production and need to reset their circadian rhythm.

To make up for lost sleep or late nights, skip the urge to sleep in. Instead, go to bed earlier for the next several nights.

THE SERENITY DETOX BATH

What you'll need: Two cups of Epson salt, 5 to 10 drops of lavender oil

Add all the ingredients to your bathwater. Use hot, but not scalding water.

Soak and relax for fifteen to twenty minutes just before bed every night. Go directly to bed after the bath.

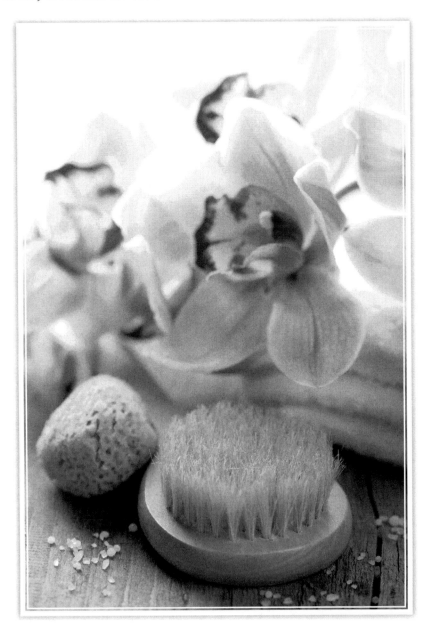

Water and Physical Movement

Water

I was reluctant to write about drinking water and exercise, but I would be remiss if I missed the opportunity to remind you of these two important elements.

Drink more water! We need it to function. You may have heard this saying, "If you feel thirsty, you are already dehydrated." You may even feel hungry when in reality it's water that your body needs. In our home, we call it boredom hunger. The kids wander around aimlessly, saying, "I'm hungry." A good test is to drink a full glass of water, wait ten minutes and then reevaluate if you are still hungry.

Drinking water throughout the day is also preferential to gulping down large glasses during a meal. We don't want to dilute stomach acid while we eat, so small sips with your meal is best.

Learning to upgrade your water is helpful if you're the type that has trouble remembering to drink water. Make it interesting by infusing your water with herbs or fruit. I add cucumber slices (anti-inflammatory), lemon slices (cleansing) and parsley or cilantro (detoxifying) to my mason jar of water.

The most common health complaints of people who are dehydrated are constipation, skin issues, headaches, muscle cramps and cravings. The amount of water each person needs depends on body weight and activity level. The general rule is to consume half your body weight in ounces. So a 160-lb person would aim to drink at least ten eight ounce glasses per day. If you exercise, or sweat throughout the day, you will need to drink more water.

Physical Movement

I had a good friend tell me once, "I hate exercise." So rather than trying to convince her to love it (like I do) or do it (because she should), I said, "Oh you're like a puddle." I went on to describe what I meant. Think of the ocean—full of life and movement as the waves crash in and around the beaches and rocks. It's an ever-changing, environmental wonder; Full of life and vitality. Now imagine that puddle is stagnant with algae, bacteria and pests. The puddle is analogous to the body that never moves—its energy stagnant and flat. Exercise and movement circulate and deliver energy and oxygen throughout the body. In Chinese medicine, movement equals health while stagnation equals disease.

Find physical movement that you enjoy. Consider your body type as a way to determine what your body needs. For example if you are prone to stiffness or chronic fatigue then running is likely to create added stress on the body and agitate you. Consider Pilates, yoga or walking as way to move energy around the body. If you are thin, weak, or more prone to anxiety, consider heavy lifting and weight training as a way to build your power and a sense of feeling grounded.

Hydration and movement will naturally create an internal environment were disease can't take hold of you. When it comes to exercise, don't be a puddle.

Seasonal Eating

SPRING FOODS	SUMMER FOODS	FALL FOODS	WINTER FOODS
Apricots	Apricots	Acorn squash	Acorn squash
Artichokes	Arugula	Arugula	Brussels sprout
Arugula	Beets	Apples	Butternut squash
Asparagus	Bell peppers*	Butternut squash	Cauliflower
Avocados*	Blackberries	Brussels Sprouts	Chestnuts
Broccoli	Blueberries	Cranberries	Clementine
Carrots *	Broccoli	Endive	Collard Greens
Cauliflower	Cantaloupe	Figs	Dates
Chicory	Cherries	Grapes	Grapefruit
Chives	Cucumbers	Hot Peppers	Kale
Collard Greens	Grapes	Jicama	Kiwi
Dandelion greens	Eggplant	Kale	Leeks*
Honeydew	Green beans	Mushrooms	Lemons*
Fennel	Hot Peppers	Parsnips*	Oranges
Grapefruit	Nectarines	Pears	Passion fruit
Green Beans	Peaches	Pomegranates	Pears
Limes	Pineapples	Pumpkin	Pineapples
Mango	Plums	Sweet potatoes	Radicchio
Peas	Raspberries	Swiss chard	Radishes
Pineapples	Summer squash	Winter squash	Rutabaga
Rhubarb	Tomatoes		Tangerines
Spinach	Watermelon		Turnips*
Spring greens	Zucchini		
Strawberries			
Sugar snap peas			
Watercress			

* Year-round foods

The rhythm of Mother Nature

Eat Seasonally

Mother Nature has created a natural rhythm of life. Too often we work against this natural order of things. All living creatures, whether human, plant or animal, must live in harmony with nature. Our survival depends on it. Birds fly south for the winter. In the fall, leaves fall from the trees making room for new growth, a rebirth in the spring.

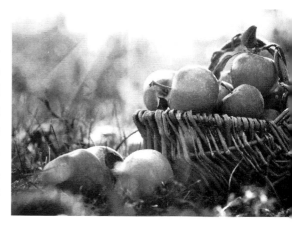

We tend to ignore our own needs to the changes that take place from one season to the next. It's not about adding an extra layer of clothing and eating the same foods. It's about eating seasonal food from our local region and building our activities around the natural rhythm of the day.

Ideally, we should be going to sleep and rising with the sun. From a dietary perspective so much of what we need during each season is provided in our food. In the summer, we tend to crave cooling foods that keep us from overheating. In the winter, we can turn to root vegetables like carrots, squash and parsnips to ground us in preparation for stormy, cold weather. And, in the spring we move to cleansing foods, like dandelion, lemons and Brussels sprouts to cleanse and detoxify the body as part of our rebirth.

Seasonal eating is hardly a new trend. Eating foods when nature produces them is what people have done naturally through most of history, before supermarkets flooded the landscape and processed foods became pervasive. Seasonal eating is also a cornerstone of ancient medical traditions, like Ayurveda, which views it as integral means to achieve balance and harmony.

Seasonal eating is a way to build meals around foods that have been freshly harvested when they are highest in nutrients. It also connects us to each other often in the form of activities that bring us together—like apple picking in autumn or soup on a cold winter day.

Self Talk

In Ayurveda, described as the "science of life", the mind is thought to be the origin of all disease. The mind creates protective patterns and belief systems that start early in childhood and shape your personality today.

As infants and toddlers, the mind is just developing and thus, rays of purity exude from the innocence of children. We move through each day in a state of wonder. But as we grow and experience hurt feelings, or compete for mommy and daddy's attention (I don't think I've had a complete conversation with my husband in years) or discover the euphoria of ice cream, we create a new, safer version of our personality.

This carries into adulthood as child-like worries of what people will think of us— Am I thin enough? Smart enough? Athletic enough? Do they like me?—This inner dialogue is interpreted as stress.

Research tells us that these emotional stresses are processed through the gut, causing the digestive process to break down first. I could write an entire book on the gut-brain connection and its impact on our health. There is enough scientific and evidence based research to support multiple books. We know the brain and the immune system continuously signal each other, often along the same pathways, which may explain how the state of mind influences our health.

For now, I am inviting you to consider how much your internal dialogue affects your body and your overall health. You are what you eat, what you digest, and what you think.

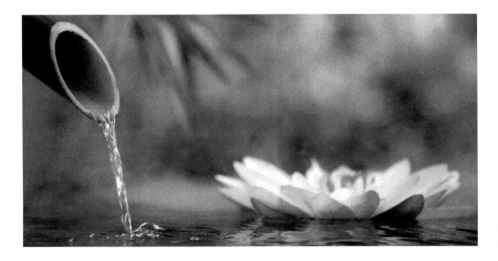

Section IV: Prevention Takeaways

Here are the three phases that you can anticipate from others in response to your new-found health—ridicule, resistance, acceptance. Be ready and stay true to yourself.

....

Failing to plan is planning to fail. Set yourself up for success.

....

Create your "safe haven" at home.
Everyone needs an environment where they feel nourished and safe around food.

....

Nutrition bridges the gap between self-care and health care.
Eat as though your life depends on it. It does.

....

Sleep your way to good health.
Lack of sleep makes you sick and fat.

....

Drink more water and move your body everyday.

....

Eat from the season.
Mother Nature has created a natural rhythm of life as your guide to dietary choices and behaviors.

....

Ask yourself today:

Is my home environment a place I feel secure and nourished?

....

Is my diet and lifestyle in sync with
the rhythm of Mother Nature?

....

Do I talk to myself in the same way I talk to those I love?

....

Am I sleeping enough?

....

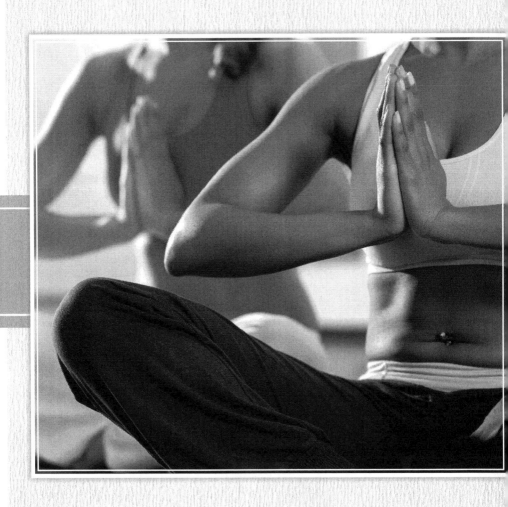

PART V: TUNING IN

Beyond The D.E.A.P. Approach

STOP COPING, START THRIVING

Most people find it easier to keep doing what they've always done rather than looking inward and searching out what they really want from life. Being authentic and walking your talk is no easy thing to do. It takes courage and conviction, both on a conscious and an unconscious level, to have the words you speak, the actions you take and the way you live your life congruent with your thoughts.

Living a life in physical and emotional pain is one challenge people face that interferes with their ability to embrace the best version of themselves. I used to describe the sensation of pain as a radio turned on too high. I wanted someone to turn down the volume so I could be more open to finding alternative solutions to my health complaints. I became reliant on pain medications to turn down the noise. Unfortunately, the medication always wore off and I was back where I started. Again and again.

Living a life in pain, with fatigue or other symptoms takes more energy and is more stressful than you realize. Taking back your personal power and being responsible for everything you do (including how you care for yourself and the food you eat) is the beginning of the breaking this vicious cycle. Eventually it become incredibly liberating and feels like a huge weight has been lifted.

Use the techniques described in this book to help you get to a place where you feel you are thriving, not surviving.

Finding your courage

I have practiced yoga for over twenty years, well sort of. I was introduced to yoga as a form of exercise at a local gym. Let's just say it was a deep stretch and I wanted to come back but it was not the "yoga" I know and practice today.

Yoga is a designed to bring more awareness to your body and your mind. However, yoga is also a system that extends far beyond the postures and far beyond the mind. I experimented over many years that followed that first introductory yoga class in different venues, different "styles" of yoga and with different teachers. Each time moved me closer to my ultimate yoga destination—yoga as a way of living within myself and beyond the mat.

My back surgery would serve to be the ultimate doorway into yoga. I woke up in the hospital following surgery alone in a room and unable to move, literally. I was paralyzed. Although it was believed to be caused by the emotional trauma of surgery, some practitioners suggested it was connected to a previous case of post-traumatic stress disorder from a vicious dog attack to my legs years prior—another example of the power of the mind-body connection. Needless to say, it was extremely frightening and very traumatic.

Recovery was slow and painful but I was determined to walk again. After a long confinement to my bed, a body brace to stabilize my hips, months of physical therapy, morphine, crutches and a walker, it was time to visit the "mat."

To prepare myself for what would be an interesting and tearful experience (more like sobbing in my case), I turned to books on spiritual wisdom including, *Yamas and Niyamas* by Deborah Adele, which helped shaped my yoga practice.

Yamas and Niyamas are the first two limbs of the eight-fold path. Adele describes the eight-fold path as basic guidelines or tenets of yoga from writings called the Yoga Sutras. The eight limbs are: Yamas (restraints), Niyamas (observances), Asana (postures), Pranayama (breath control), Pratahara (sense withdrawal), Dharana (concentrataion), Dhyana (meditation) and Samadhi (state of unity).

The first yama is Ahimsa, which means nonviolence. Initially, I thought this meant killing or doing physical harm. However I now understand this as more subtle implications to nonviolence like being harsh with myself, unkind to others, verbally exploding at my spouse or children, or living in fear. Adele describes the difference between the fear that keeps us alive (instinctual/survival) and the fear that keeps us from living. She believes fear creates violence through greed, control and insecurity.

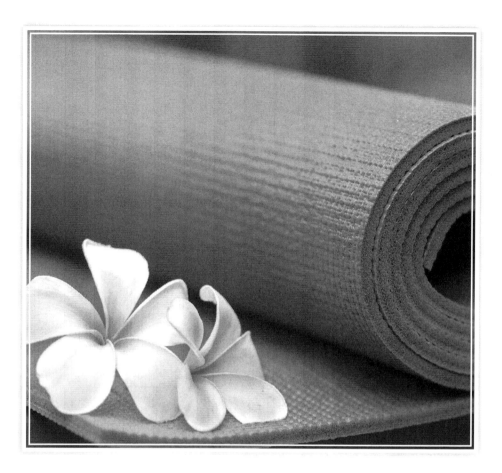

Finding courage is spite of my fear was critical to my healing. "Courage," she says," is not the absence of fear, but the ability to be afraid without being paralyzed."

The Niyama that shook my world was self-study, as in knowing ourselves and studying what drives us. Ultimately this tenet invites you to release false and limiting self-perception that your ego has imposed on you. When you begin to unravel your own belief system, painful emotions are often released in the process (this explains the crying).

I took the meaning of self-study even further by exploring my beliefs around health and wellness. As a former recreational triathlete, I thought I had a good grasp of what living a healthy life consisted of: exercise and whole grains. But I was looking at the definition of health as a way to analyze and fix everything but still keep control. In other words, a new diet that must be the answer but one that still allows me to eat the foods I am not willing to give up. We tend to keep things the way we like them, making small adjustments to demonstrate effort (or willingness to change) but maintaining full control over old beliefs and patterns.

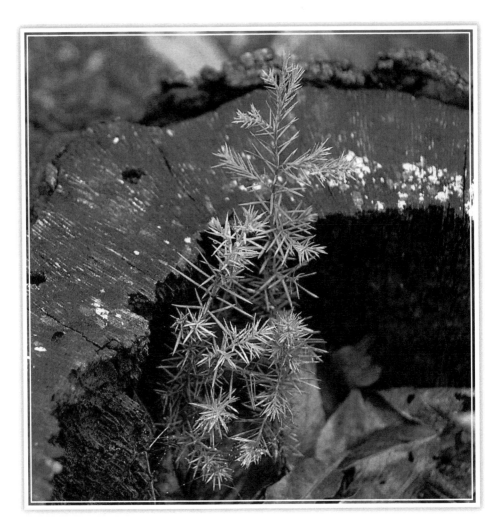

Other forms of self-study include meditation but not in the way you might think. Meditation invites you to steady the mind and return to the breath. In this way, you can shift your belief that the answers to your questions reside inside of you, rather than externally. The Buddhists remind us to have a beginner's mind—to know that we don't know. As Adele so eloquently says, "It is this stance of humility that opens the door to learning and revelation."

Keep in mind there is no right or wrong way to explore yoga, meditation, mindfulness or any practice that invites you to discover more about yourself. I simply share my experience and invite you to find one that resonates with you so that you too can explore the possibility of living your best life.

Find something that serves as a constant reminder to "never give up."

The pursuit of health and happiness

Happiness

Noun: A state of being

Synonyms: pleasure, contentment, satisfaction, cheerfulness, joy

Shawn Achor, author of *The Happiness Advantage*, uses the definition of happiness from the ancient Greek meaning "it's the joy we feel striving toward our potential." I like to point out that this is beyond "pleasure." Pleasure is a momentary feeling that comes from something external—a good meal, the stock market going up or making love. Happiness is a state of mind and a reflection of our internal satisfaction with our life. It doesn't happen once a week. We don't arrive at happiness. We have to strive for our life's purpose and happiness and joy is the journey that way.

I see nutrition in a very similar or complementary way. It nourishes us on our journey to pursue our life's purpose. If the food we eat and the environment we live in holds us back, creating pain and suffering, then our journey to our life's purpose becomes weighted and cloudy. Having the "cheat" meal of the week is the perfect example of seeking pleasure, not living in joy. When we learn to postpone joy from our food, we are programed to feel a sense of suffering until that point. I think that's an unhealthy relationship with food.

Your happiness also comes from how your brain processes your life. It does not have to be driven by our environment. Happiness can be a choice. Perhaps, this explains why Pharrell Williams' song "Happy" is the most-played song, topping Billboard's Radio Songs chart for eight weeks, the longest lead on the chart in 2014. We all want to feel happy.

Even our success does not equal happiness. Success is a moving target. For example, if your goal is to loose weight, when you reach this goal you will expect to be happy. Instead you change your definition of happiness because you will quickly realize your weight goal is not happiness, now you want better skin, or a new house. Your definition of happiness or the success you associate with happiness keeps moving.

Daniel Gilbert, Ph.D., Harvard psychologist and author of *Stumbling on Happiness,* says, "We're such strangers to ourselves." I think this is so true. We have lost touch with our authentic self and spend very little time reflecting on the very things that make us feel happy—striving toward our potential.

HEALTH

Noun: the state of being free from illness or injury.

Synonyms: well-being, healthiness, fitness, good condition, fine

Stop chasing health. It's right in front of you. You don't need a program or a diet to get it. What you may need is a guide to educate you on how to see it and how to help you identify what your purpose in life is. When you pursue your purpose—what lights you up—you are more likely to eat foods that nourish your body.

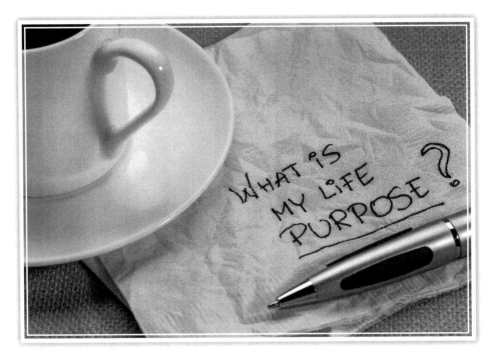

The definition of health implies that the absence of disease (or illness) is health. If you consider that the cause of disease is unique to the individual, then the solution to achieve or regain one's state of health is also unique. Health does not happen in the doctor's office. It happens in your kitchen. It happens in your home. It happens in your community.

We receive advice and information about our health from every direction. We have come to rely on external sources to find the answer to internal problems. We read books (thank you), we follow blogs, do all kinds of research—often living in an endless search for "the answer." Instead, if we shift our focus on what's happening inside our body and our mind, we often uncover the root cause of disease or imbalance better than anyone else.

I believe food and lifestyle fall into two categories: nourishment or depletion. There is no in between. That doesn't mean that things like sweets, coffee or late nights always fall into the depletion category as you might assume. Envision these two scenarios: You're sitting on your back porch with a cup of coffee on beautiful fall morning with your favorite book or enjoying a conversation with your spouse before the children rise. Now, imagine yourself rushing out the door, late for work, only to arrive at a very long line at the Dunkin Donuts drive-through where you wait for coffee you "need" to get you through the day at the job you hate. I think you get the point.

BUILDING YOUR HEALTH AND HAPPINESS MUSCLE

We should be the happiest and healthiest nation. This is an exciting time. But, instead we are depressed, anxious, suffering, and chronically ill. We are yearning for something bigger than our day-to day grind. We are starving for something beyond what we are doing every day. Our purpose.

Health and happiness is part of self-care. Daily habits like brushing your teeth are automatic. You can also create health and happiness habits:

- Identify things you are grateful for. What you focus on gets stronger.

- Practice optimism.

- Make of list of experiences that bring you joy. Look for the common thread in those activities to see what fills your bucket.

- Stop exercising to loose weight. Exercise because you love your body not because you hate it.

- Practice stillness. Breathe. Start with five minutes to rest and reset your brain from the busy setting.

Accept yourself as you are.
Nourish yourself in a way that makes you feel good,
not in way that seeks to change who you really are.

Choose health and happiness.

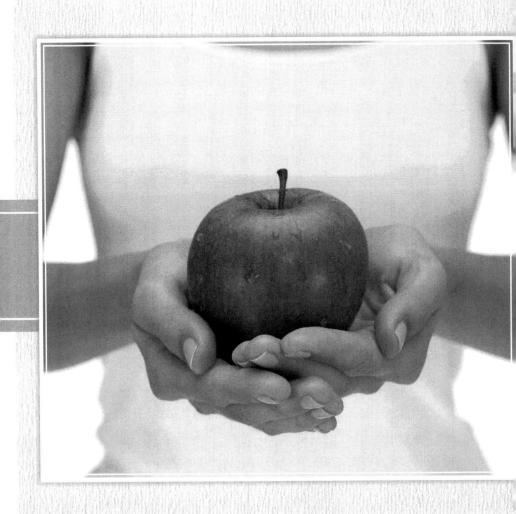

Learn More about Health & Nutrition

WE NEED MORE HEALTH COACHES AND HOLISTIC PRACTITIONERS

People are struggling despite their efforts to resolve their chronic health condition. Many people visit multiple doctors, specialists and nutritionists in search for the answer to their health concerns only to leave even more frustrated and confused. We must move away the band-aid approach to health. We need more practitioners who want to explore the root cause of disease and listen to the individual that is suffering. So often, the information needed to heal comes from the individual in pain. People need guidance and support. There are so many reputable and comprehensive programs available today whether you're interested in personal growth or a complete change of career. All programs are online/distance learning. Here is a brief overview of some of the programs I recommend. As always, I suggest you do your own research on the programs mentioned below and decide which, if any, are a good fit for you.

INSTITUTE FOR INTEGRATIVE NUTRITION (IIN) ™

IIN offers a Certified Holistic Health Coach program where you will learn over 100 dietary theories that will help you customize dietary protocols for clients based upon their unique bio-individuality. The benefit of this open-minded and individualized approach is that you will learn 'how to think' not 'what to think.' The teaching faculty is nothing short of amazing, including Andrew Weil, M.D., Mark Hyman, M.D., Deepak Chopra, M.D. and many more. IIN does not teach the clinical approach to nutrition so you will not learn to run lab tests or address more complex health conditions with this certification alone. But don't underestimate the value of the counseling education at IIN. The teaching model addresses all aspects of health, like relationships, finances, spirituality and environment as your "primary foods ™" and the food we eat as "secondary foods." You will also receive the necessary business tools to build a successful career and the connections you will make to students around the world is priceless.

As part of the IIN Ambassador program, I am able to offer scholarships toward your tuition at any time. Upon enrollment, ask for the *Ambassador Savings Offer* and give them my name. If there's another savings offer going on of equal or greater value, you will automatically receive that scholarship.

To learn more visit www.integrativenutrition.com

Functional Diagnostic Nutrition (FDN)

The FDN certification course is an intense online course that gets incredibly clinical about finding the root cause of health issues using top quality lab work. They train you to become a "health detective", focusing intently on the many facets of digestive health including identifying leaky gut or dysbiosis and pathogens (bad baceteria/parasites/yeast/mold), while also training you to identify liver and kidney issues, and all manners of hormonal imbalances.

FDN can help you understand how to use and customize supplement protocols while teaching you which labs to use/run to help clients heal from the root cause. There is significant support on how to interpret lab results and client cases through the Medical Director program. FDN provides you with a step-by-step method to engage your clients and patients in the healing process so that the clients actually get the information they need and the results they want. By gaining a complete understanding of the functions of the body, you will be able to address the root cause of dysfunction.

To learn more, visit: www.functionaldiagnosticnutrition.com

Certified Clinical Nutritionist (CCN)

The Clinical Nutrition Certification Board (CNCB) is an agency, which provides professional training, examination and certification for health care organizations, including state license/certification examinations. Its an in-depth program requires some prerequisite science classes before enrolling, depending on your prior education. They provide a national board certification to practice nutrition in all states. If you are looking to be certified nationally as a nutritionist, this program provides that.

To learn more, visit: www.cncb.org

Institute for Functional Medicine (IFM)

IFM's certification program is a comprehensive, clinical training for assessment, treatment, prevention, and management of patients with complex, chronic disease. After successful completion of written examinations following the completion of AFMCP and the six Advanced Practice Modules, the clinician is then certified as a functional medicine practitioner.

To learn more, visit: www.functionalmedicine.org

Holistic Nutrition Lab

Holistic Nutrition Lab differs from other functional medicine and nutrition training because its Founder, Andrea Nakayama, provides a forum where anatomy and physiology are being looked at through the lens of nutrition. In many functional training programs there is a strong focus on the theoretical. Andrea is a functional nutritionist with the clinical experience to give you practical advice and guidance. She offers case studies and protocols that apply to specific conditions which help you become an effective, efficient health practitioner. If you are looking for a background in the fundamental basics of the body and how food affects your health, you will benefit from this program.

To learn more, visit: www.holisticnutritionlab.com

BioIndividual Nutrition Institute

BioIndividual Nutrition is the science and clinical application of personalized diet and nutrition. The BioIndividual Nutrition Institute empowers clinicians who understand that most chronic health conditions have underlying imbalances and require an individualized approach. Their BioIndividual Nutrition training program provides the necessary tools to customize diet and nutrition protocols and a technology platform that revolutionizes how health practitioners support their patients/clients success. They aim to advance the efficacy of individualizing food, special diets, and nutrient needs for the prevention and healing of disease. It is led by a practicing nutrition consultant and includes business and practice tools based on more than a decade of clinical experience. Graduates become Certified BioIndividual Nutrition Practitioners and have the option of an additional certification course that specializing in Nutrition for Children, Autism, ADHD and other Special Needs.

To learn more, visit: www.bioindividualnutrition.com

Specialized Training Programs

Living on Live Food: Raw Chef Teacher Certification

Whether your looking for a career in raw food or just interested in learning more for yourself, Alissa has been eating and teaching the raw food lifestyle since 1986. She was one of the first to begin a Certification Program in this field. This four-day, hands-on training takes place in Gloucester, MA and includes a full day of advanced raw food preparation with restaurant chef and co-author of *Raw Food for Everyone*, Leah Dubois. Certified students go on to teach Level One and Two classes, open restaurants, become personal chefs, write books, consult and more. Alissa Cohen's Level 3 Certification course is designed to open up a whole new world for you by giving you the knowledge and training to become a certified Living on Live Food Chef, Instructor and Teacher. Both newcomers and experienced participants feel comfortable in Alissa's class. You will learn about food preparation and nutrition, but also gain the tools to inspire others along their wellness path.

To learn more, visit: www.alissacohen.com

Certified Gluten Practitioner

The Certified Gluten Practitioner (CGP) program is a comprehensive practitioner education available for understanding non-celiac gluten sensitivity (NCGS) and celiac disease (CD). The program presents an in-depth understanding of the causes of non-celiac gluten sensitivity (NCGS) and celiac disease (CD) to help health care and nutrition practitioners (and their staff) diagnose, treat and educate people about these disorders. It is ideal for healthcare practitioners who want to learn more about helping patients suffering with gluten-related disorders.

To learn more, visit: www.thedr.com

Environmental Toxins

Environmental toxicity is something that touches each and every health condition—from weight gain and diabetes, to thyroid disease, infertility, and cancers. Lara Adler offers different levels of training for Health & Wellness Professionals who are seeking to better understand the links between chemicals & human health. Courses give practitioners the tools to better serve and support their client's goals, and so they themselves can live more in alignment with their healthy lifestyles. A core of all trainings is taking dense, often intimidating and overwhelming, information and breaking it down in easy to understand language, and offering real world, practical solutions that can be implemented right away.

To learn more, visit: www.laraadler.com

Institute of Nutritional Leadership

The Institute of Nutritional Leadership (INL) is led by Dr. Joshua Axe, D.C., C.N.S., and is designed to help individuals who are passionate about nutrition and wellness to turn their knowledge into a successful business. While open to anyone with a passion for teaching others about nutrition, this program primarily draws, and is ideal for, health coaches, chiropractors, nutritionists, fitness instructors, medical professionals and health enthusiasts who want to influence a wider audience. This 8-week health coaching program, which includes nutrition, healing foods, plant-based medicine, marketing strategies, branding, content creation and more, is delivered online with two weekly training classes. INL also offers a membership forum that houses the audio, video and transcripts of the course, as well as, a private social media forum for students from around the world to connect and collaborate throughout the program.

To learn more, please visit: http://my.draxe.com/inl-welcome

References

1 Libby, P. (2006) Inflammation and cardiovascular disease mechanisms. The American Journal of Clinical Nutrition. Feb;83 (2):456S-460S.

2 Weinhold, B., "Epigenetics: The Science of Change." *Environmental Health Perspective.* Mar 2006; 114(3): A160–A167

3 Fasano, A., "Leaky gut and Autoimmune Disease." Clinical Reviews in Allergy and Immunology. 2012 Feb;42(1):71-8. doi: 10.1007/s12016-011-8291-x.

4 Curtis, L.T., Patel, K. "Nutritional and environmental approaches to preventing and treating autism and attention deficit hyperactivity disorder (ADHD)". *Journal of Alternative and Complimentary Medicine.* 2008. Jan-Feb; 14(1): 79-85

5 Julie Matthews. Nourishing Hope for Autism: Nutrition and Diet for Healing our Children. 2008. P. 79

6 Ibid

7 Wester P.O., Magnesium. *American Journal of Clinical Nutrition.* 1987;45:1305-12.

8 Saris N.E., Mervaala E., Karppanen H., Khawaja J.A., Lewenstam A., "Magnesium: An Update on Physiological, Clinical, and Analytical Aspects." *The International Journal of Clinical Chemistry.* 2000;294:1-26

9 Shankar, A.H., Prasad A.S., "Zinc and Immune Function: The Biological Basis of Altered Resistance to Infection." *American Journal of Clinicial Nutrition.* 1998;68 (suppl):447S–63S.

10 Prasad AS, Clinical Manifestations of Zinc Deficiency, Annual Review of Nutrition. 1985;5:341-63.

11 Rannem T1, Ladefoged K, Hylander E, Hegnhøj J, Staun M., "Selenium depletion in patients with gastrointestinal diseases: Are there any predictive factors?" *Scandinavian Journal of Gastroenterology.* 1998. Oct;33(10):1057-61

12 Thomson CD1, Chisholm A, McLachlan SK, Campbell JM., "Brazil nuts: An effective way to improve selenium status." *American Journal of Clinical Nutrition.* 2008. Feb;87(2):379-84.

13 Chowdhury R, Warnakula S, Kunutsor S, et al. Association of Dietary, Circulating, and Supplement Fatty Acids With Coronary Risk: A Systematic Review and Meta-analysis. Annals of Internal Medicine. Published online March 18 2014

14 Loomis, Jr., Howard F. Introduction to Enzymes: They Key to Health. Vol. 1 The Fundamentals. (Century Nutrition Publication. 2007), xxiii

15 Ciafalo V, et al., Safety evaluation of an alpha-amylase enzyme preparation derived from the archaeal order Thermococcales as expressed in Pseudomonas fluorescens biovar I. *Regul. Toxicol. Pharmacol.* 37:149 2003.

16 Coenen TM, et al. Safety evaluation of a lactase enzyme preparation derived from Kluyveromyces lactis. *Food Chem. Toxicol.* 38:671. 2000.

17 Lissau BG, et al. Safey evaluation of a fungal pectinesterase enzyme preparation and its use in food. *Food Addit. Contam.* 15:627. 1998.

18 Coenen TM, et al. Safety evaluation of amino peptidase enzyme preparation derived from Aspergillus niger. *Food Chem. Toxicol.* 36:781. 1998

19 Bergman, A, et al. An overview of the safety evaluation of the Thermomyces lanuginosus xylanase enzyme (SP 628) and the Aspergillus aculeatus xylanase enzyme (SP 578). *Food Addit. Contam.* 14:389. 1997

20 Champagne ET. Low gastric hydrochloric acid secretion and mineral bioavailability. Adv Exp Med Biol. 1989;249:173-84.21

21 Gibson PR, Shepherd SJ. Evidence-based dietary management of functional gastrointestinal symptoms: The FODMAP approach. *J Gastroenterol Hepatol.* 2010;25(2):252-258.22

22 Smith MR, Eastman CI; Shift work: health, performance and safety problems, traditional countermeasures, and innovative management strategies to reduce circadian misalignment. Nat Sci Sleep. 2012 Sep 27;4:111-32. doi: 10.2147/NSS. S10372. Print 2012.

23 Sigurdardottir LG, Valdimarsdottir UA, Fall K, et al; Circadian disruption, sleep loss, and prostate cancer risk: a systematic review of epidemiologic studies. Cancer Epidemiol Biomarkers Prev. 2012 Jul;21(7):1002-11. doi: 10.1158/1055-9965.EPI-12-0116. Epub 2012 May 7.

24 Haus E, Sackett-Lundeen L, Smolensky MH; Rheumatoid arthritis: circadian rhythms in disease activity, signs and symptoms, and rationale for chronotherapy with corticosteroids and other medications. Bull NYU Hosp Jt Dis. 2012;70 Suppl 1:3-10.

25 Olney JW. Brain Lesions, Obesity, and Other Disturbances in Mice Treated With Monosodium Glutamate. *Science,* 1969, 164: 719-21.

26 Block, MD, Russell. Excitotoxins: The Taste That Kills You. (Health Press, 1996).

27 Hilary Parker. A sweet problem: Princeton researchers find that high-fructose corn syrup prompts considerably more weight gain. Princeton University. 2010 March 22.

28 Jennifer K. Nelson R.D.,L.D. What is high-fructose corn syrup? What are the health concerns? Mayo Clinic. 2012 September 27.

29 Bijal Patel, Robert Schutte, Peter Sporns, Jason Doyle, Lawrence Jewel, Richard N Fedorak (2002) "Potato glycoalkaloids adversely affect intestinal permeability and aggravate inflammatory bowel disease." Inflamm Bowel Dis. 2002 Sep; 8(5):340-6. PMID: 12479649

30 An Apparent Relation of Nightshades (Solanaceae) to Arthritis http://www.noarthritis. com/research.htm Journal of Neurological and Orthopedic Medical Surgery (1993) 12:227-231.

31 http://www.iom.edu/Reports/2011/ Relieving-Pain-in-America-A-Blueprint-for-Transforming-Prevention-Care-Education-Research.aspx

32 Martinez J1, Lewi JE. ,"An unusual case of gynecomastia associated with soy product consumption." *American College of Endocrinology and American Association of Clinical Endocrinologists.* 2008. May-Jun;14(4):415-8.

33 "Soy Diet Prompts Prisoner Lawsuit." The Washington Times. February 28, 2012. Accessed September 9, 2014. http://www. washingtontimes.com/news/2012/feb/28/soy-diet-prompts-prisoners-lawsuit/?page=all

34 "Gluten: What You Don't Know Might Kill You." Dr. Mark Hyman. The Huffington Post. Updated 2011. Accessed September 9, 2014 http://www. huffingtonpost.com/dr-mark-hyman/gluten-what-you-dont-know_b_379089.html

35 Farrell RJ, Kelly CP. Celiac sprue. *New England Journal of Medicine.* 2002 Jan 17;346(3):180-8. Review.

36 Margutti P, Delunardo F, Ortona E. Autoantibodies associated with psychiatric disorders. *Curr Neurovasc Res.* 2006 May;3(2):149-57. Review.

37 Ludvigsson JF, Reutfors J, Osby U, Ekbom A, Montgomery SM. Coeliac disease and risk of mood disorders—a general population-based cohort study. *J Affect Disord.*2007 Apr;99(1-3):117-26. Epub 2006 Oct 6.

38 Ludvigsson JF, Osby U, Ekbom A, Montgomery SM. Coeliac disease and risk of schizophrenia and other psychosis: a general population cohort study. *Scand J Gastroenterol.* 2007 Feb;42(2):179-85.

39 Hu WT, Murray JA, Greenaway MC, Parisi JE, Josephs KA. Cognitive impairment and celiac disease. *Arch Neurol.* 2006 Oct;63(10):1440-6.

40 Bushara KO. Neurologic presentation of celiac disease. *Gastroenterology.* 2005 Apr;128(4 Suppl 1):S92-7. Review.

41 Millward C, Ferriter M, Calver S, Connell-Jones G. Gluten- and casein-free diets for autistic spectrum disorder. *Cochrane Database Syst Rev.* 2004;(2):CD003498. Review.

42 Green PH, Jabri B. Coeliac disease. *Lancet.* 2003 Aug 2;362(9381):383-91. Review.

43 Davis, M.D. William Wheat Belly. Rodale; 1 edition (August 30, 2011)

44 Samsel, A. and Seneff, S. Glyphosate, pathways to modern diseases II: Celiac sprue and gluten intolerance. Interdisciplinary Toxicology. Dec 2013; 6(4): 159–184. Published online Dec 2013. doi: 10.2478/intox-2013-0026

45 Video: Jeffrey Smith interviews Dr. Stephanie Seneff about Glyphosate

46 Samsel, A. and Seneff, S., Glyphosate's Suppression of Cytochrome P450 Enzymes and Amino Acid Biosynthesis by the Gut Microbiome: Pathways to Modern Diseases. *Entropy* 2013, 15(4), 1416-1463; doi:10.3390/e15041416

47 Ibid

48 Séralini GE1, Clair E, Mesnage R, Gress S, Defarge N, Malatesta M, Hennequin D, de Vendômois JS. Long term toxicity of a Roundup herbicide and a Roundup-tolerant genetically modified maize. Food and Chemical Toxicology. 2012 Nov;50(11):4221-31. doi: 10.1016/j.fct.2012.08.005. Epub 2012 Sep 19.

49 Aris A1, Leblanc S. Maternal and fetal exposure to pesticides associated to genetically modified foods in Eastern Townships of Quebec, Canada. *Reproductive Toxicology.* 2011 May;31(4):528-33. doi: 10.1016/j.reprotox.2011.02.004. Epub 2011 Feb 18.

50 See note 44 above.

51 See note 44 above.

52 Video: Jeffrey Smith interviews Dr. Stephanie Seneff about Glyphosate

53 Ruthann A. Rudel, Janet M. Gray, Connie L. Engel, Teresa W. Rawsthorne, Robin E. Dodson, Janet M. Ackerman, Jeanne Rizzo, Janet L. Nudelman, Julia Green Brody. Food Packaging and Bisphenol A and Bis (2-Ethyhexyl) Phthalate Exposure: Findings from a Dietary Intervention. Environmental Health Perspective. 2011 July 1; 119(7): 914–920. Published online 2011 March 30. doi: 10.1289/ehp.1003170

54 Ibid

55 Carwile, Jenny L., MPH, Ye, Xiaoyun, MS, Zhou, Xiaoliu, MS, Dr. Antonia M. Calafat, PhD, and Dr. Karin B. Michels, ScD, PhD, Canned Soup Consumption and Urinary Bisphenol A: A Randomized Crossover Trial. JAMA. Nov 23, 2011; 306(20): 2218–2220. doi: 10.1001/jama.2011.1721

56 Leisa-Maree L. Toms, Andreas Sjödin, Fiona Harden, Peter Hobson, Richard Jones, Emily Edenfield, and Jochen F. Mueller. Serum Polybrominated Diphenyl Ether (PBDE) Levels Are Higher in Children (2–5 Years of Age) than in Infants and Adults. Environ Health Perspect. Sep 2009; 117(9): 1461–1465. Published online May 6, 2009. doi: 10.1289/ehp.0900596

57 Ye X, Bishop AM, Reidy JA, Needham LL, Calafat AM (2006). Parabens as urinary biomarkers of exposure in humans. Environmental Health Perspectives114: 1843-1846.

58 Gray, J (2008). State of the Evidence: The Connection between Breast Cancer and the Environment. San Francisco, CA: The Breast Cancer Fund.

59 Byford JR, Shaw LE, Drew MGB, Pope GS, Sauer MJ, Darbre PD (2002). Oestrogenic activity of parabens in MCF7 human breast cancer cells. Journal of Steroid Biochemistry & Molecular Biology 80:49-60

60 Houlihan J, Brody C, Schwan B (2002). Not Too Pretty: Phthalates, Beauty Products and the FDA. Available online: http://www.safecosmetics.org/downloads/NotTooPretty_report.pdf. Accessed August 21, 2008.

61 Manori JS, et al. (2000). Urinary levels of seven phthalate metabolites in a human reference population. Environmental Health Perspectives. 112(3): 331-338.

62 Swann SH, et al.(2005). Decrease in Anogenital Distance among Male Infants with Prenatal Phthalate Exposure. Environmental Health Perspectives, 113: 1056-1061. Available online: http://www.ehponline.org/members/2005/8100/8100.pdf. Accessed July 24, 2008.

63 January 11, 2012 *Fabric Softeners Contain Toxic Chemicals.* By Selena Keegan, www.naturalnews.com

64 Lanphear BP, Vorhees CV, Bellinger DC (2005) Protecting Children from Environmental Toxins. PLoS Med 2(3): e61. doi:10.1371/journal.pmed.0020061

65 Perlmutter, MD, David. http://www.drperlmutter.com/eat/foods-that-contain-gluten/

66 Sturniolo GC1, Di Leo V, Ferronato A, D'Odorico A, D'Incà R., Zinc supplementation tightens "leaky gut" in Crohn's disease. Inflamm Bowel Dis. 2001 May;7(2):94-8

67 Weston A. Price Foundation. www.westonaprice.org

68 "Gelatin treats ulcer." *Medical News Today*. Aug 22 2006. http://www.medicalnewstoday.com/releases/50126.php

69 Russell, A. L. "Glycoaminoglycan (GAG) deficiency in protective barrier as an underlying, primary cause of ulcerative colitis, Crohn's disease interstitial cystitis and possibly Reiter's syndrome."Medical Hypotheses. April 1999 Vol. 52; 4. P 297-301.

70 Bethesda M. A Closer Look at Ayurvedic Medicine. Focus on Complementary and Alternative Medicine. National Center for Complementary and Alternative Medicine, US National Institutes of Health, US National Institutes of Health. 2006;XII(4)

71 Asokan S1, Rathan J, Muthu MS, Rathna PV, Emmadi P; Raghuraman; Chamundeswari. Effect of oil pulling on Streptococcus mutans count in plaque and saliva using Dentocult SM Strip mutans test: a randomized, controlled, triple-blind study. J Indian Soc Pedod Prev Dent. 2008 Mar;26(1):12-7.

72 Ni CH, Hou WH, Kao CC, Et Al. The anxiolytic effect of aromatherapy on patients awaiting ambulatory surgery: a randomized controlled trial. Evid Based Complement Alternat Med. 2013;2013:927419.

73 Hodge NS, McCarthy MS, Pierce RM. A prospective randomized study of the effectiveness of aromatherapy for relief of postoperative nausea and vomiting. J Perianesth Nurs. 2014;29(1):5-11.

74 Jeena K, Liju VB, Kuttan R. Antioxidant, anti-inflammatory and antinociceptive activities of essential oil from ginger. Indian J Physiol Pharmacol. 2013;57(1):51-62.

75 Oboh G, Olasehinde TA, Ademosun AO. Essential oil from lemon peels inhibit key enzymes linked to neurodegenerative conditions and pro-oxidant induced lipid peroxidation. J Oleo Sci. 2014;63(4):373-381.

76 El-Sherbiny GM, El Sherbiny. The effect of Commiphora molmol (Myrrh) in treatment of Trichomoniasis vaginalis infection. Iran Red Crescent Med J. 2011;13(7):480-486.

77 Su S, Wang T, Duan JA, et al. Anti-inflammatory and analgesic activity of different extracts of *Commiphora myrrha*. J Ethnopharmacol. 2011;134(2):251-258.

78 Saeed S, Tariq P. Antibacterial activity of oregano (*Origanum vulgare* Linn.) against gram positive bacteria. Pak J Pharm Sci. 2009;22(4):421-424.

79 Force M, Sparks WS, Ronzio RA. Inhibition of enteric parasites by emulsified oil of oregano in vivo. Phytotherapy Research. 2000;14:213-214.

80 al-Sereiti MR, Abu-Amer KM, Sen P. Pharmacology of rosemary (Rosmarinus officinalis Linn.) and its therapeutic potentials. Indian J Exp Biol. 1999;37(2):124-130.

81 Ludvigsson JF, Montgomery SM, Ekbom A, Brandt L, Granath F. Small-intestinal histopathology and mortality risk in celiac disease. *JAMA*. 2009 Sep 16;302(11):1171-8.

Meet the Author

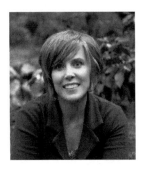

After years of struggling with fibromyalgia, chronic fatigue, severe degenerative arthritis, chronic pain syndrome and a myriad of other ailments, Kathleen made it her personal mission to spread the word about the power of healthy food and the astounding ways in which food can positively transform your life. Her knowledge of nutrition has been carefully developed through years of both professional and self-study.

Kathleen prides herself on a wide range of nutritional wisdom, food savvy and self-care techniques. She is trained in Functional Nutrition, Bio-Individual Nutrition, and is a Certified Health and Nutrition Coach. She has specialized training in the biomedical approaches and supplemental interventions to autism. Kathleen is also professionally trained as a raw food chef. She is board certified by the American Association of Drugless Practitioners.

Kathleen serves as the President and Chair of the Board of Directors for Rhode Island Parent Information Network (RIPIN), a non-profit agency that serves over 40,000 individuals with special health care needs in the areas of health, education and advocacy.

As a gluten-free lifestyle expert, Kathleen is also the Branch Manager of the Gluten Intolerance Group of Northern Rhode Island, a local branch for the national non-profit organization with a vision of support, acceptance, and respect for all persons living with gluten-related disorders, including celiac and non-celiac gluten sensitivity (NCGS).

Kathleen proudly leads the Northern Rhode Island Chapter for the Weston A. Price Foundation (WAPF), which is dedicated to restoring nutrient-dense foods to the human diet through education, research and activism.

Kathleen believes in the importance of giving back to her community through service. She is the Founder of Rhode to Health (www.rhodetohealth.com), a community-based resource dedicated to teaching and empowering others in Rhode Island (and beyond), to embrace the self-care model to dig us out of the healthcare crisis. She also sits on a number of local advisory committees that support wellness programs in public schools and chronic healthcare in Rhode Island.

Kathleen lives in Lincoln RI with her husband and three young boys.

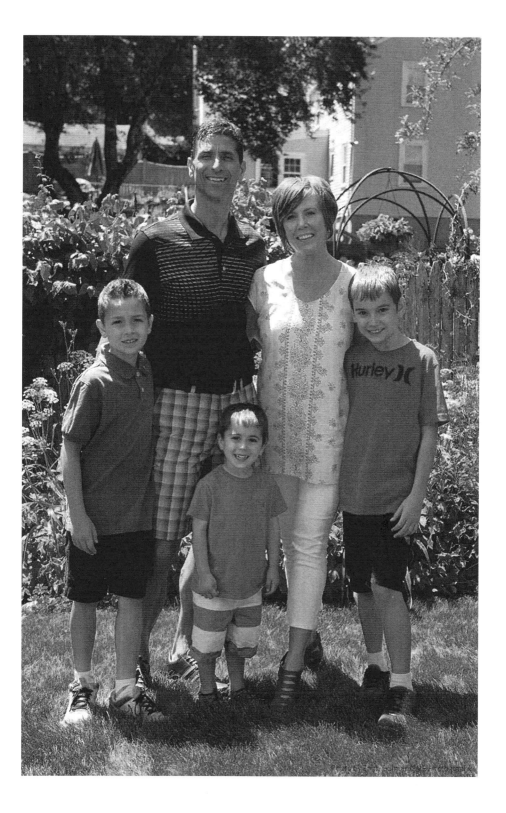

About the Cover

The eyes are the window to the soul

The eyes reveal so much about the health of the body, mind and spirit. From physical signs of internal inflammation to the emotions of joy and excitement, the eyes tell a story of who we are, how we feel and what we believe.

Diagnostically, we can "see" signs of internal inflam- mation and food allergies in red, swollen, itchy eyes. Besides inadequate sleep and fatigue that are also known to cause dark under-eye circles directly or indirectly, dark circles together with sunken eyelids can also be the result of poor nutrition. Thinning or the loss of hair on the eyebrow is a telltale sign of thyroid issues, while certain eye diseases, like cata- racts and macular degeneration, can be reduced by specific nutrients like B6, vitamin C, omega-3 fatty acids and lutein (antioxidant).

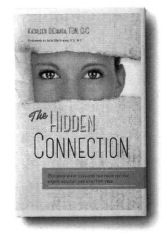

Symbolically, the eye is considered a universal symbol representing spiritual sight, in- ner vision, higher knowledge, conscious awareness, and insight. The physical eye has a pupil symbolizing we are pupils (students) in a universe (university). I believe when we move through life as a student, open and ready to learn and grow, we have our best experience on earth.

Throughout history, eye iconography has been used in different cultures and reli- gions. The Hebrew literature talks of the watchful eyes of the Lord looking over all cre- ation. The Egyptians have the Eye of Horus that symbolizes protection, good health and royal power. In Hinduism, there are references to Lord Shiva's "third eye," and in Buddhism, the Buddha is known as "Eye of the world". In Christianity, the triangle enclosing the eye is symbolic of the Holy Trinity, while the rays of light around it repre- sent divinity and spiritual illumination.

I believe we are all the eyes of the universe.

Notes

28630999R00106

Made in the USA
Middletown, DE
22 January 2016